SILENT SCARS OF HEALING HANDS

ORAL HISTORIES OF JAPANESE AMERICAN DOCTORS IN WORLD WAR II DETENTION CAMPS

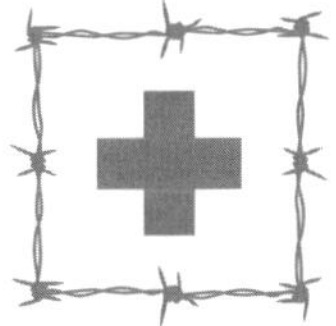

by Naomi Hirahara and
Gwenn M. Jensen

A California Civil Liberties Public Education Program project of the Japanese American Medical Association, in conjunction with the Japanese American National Museum and the UCLA Asian American Studies Center as part of the Michi Nishiura and Walter Weglyn Multicultural Publication Series.

APPLEWOOD BOOKS

This book was published originally under the copyright of Dr. Gordon H. Sasaki, MD, with the support of the Japanese American Medical Association (JAMA) in 2004, and was gifted to the Japanese American National Museum (JANM) in 2005. If you would like to donate to JAMA, please go to www.jamasocal.org

Published by Applewood Books, an imprint of Arcadia Publishing.

Charleston, South Carolina

For a complete list of books currently available, please visit us at www.applewoodbooks.com

Library of Congress Control Number: 2025943822

ISBN 978-1-4290-0603-3

Printed in the USA

So that's the only thing positive I got out of camp, is [that] *I learned to listen to hearts and lungs.*

—Mary (Sakaguchi) Oda, MD

FOREWORD

I am confident that the late Michi Nishiura Weglyn would have welcomed *Silent Scars of Healing Hands*, the newest addition to this multicultural book series bearing her and her husband Walter's name. During my frequent postal, telephonic, and in-person communications with Michi between 1974 and 1999, she invariably brought up matters of sickness and health for extended discussion. Although she suffered during this interval from a variety of afflictions, culminating in the cancer that took her life, she typically steered our conversation away from herself and toward the health problems of mutual friends and associates as well as me and my family members.

Ironically, one subject I never recall being brought up in our talks, except in passing, was the medical care she and other Japanese American inmates received while incarcerated in U.S. government detention camps during World War II. Had Michi been stricken with tuberculosis as a teenager at the Gila Relocation Center in south-central Arizona's desert instead of during her postwar resettlement in the eastern United States, the situation might well have been quite different. Surely having been under the close and constant care of Japanese American doctors such as those in this book would have called forth from her many poignant, interesting, and significant memories.

Michi Weglyn was vitally interested in the healing process of righting wrongs, whether those wrongs affected individuals or nation-states. I am convinced that her primary motivation for writing her classic 1976 book, *Years of Infamy: The Untold Story of America's*

Concentration Camps, was to heal America rather than simply to indict it for illegally depriving one of its racial-ethnic groups of life, liberty, and the pursuit of happiness. Were Michi still alive, *Silent Scars of Healing Hands* would be doubly welcomed by her, for it is both an untold story about the camp experience and one whose protagonists are healers.

Arthur A. Hansen
Series Editor
Center for Oral and Public History,
California State University, Fullerton

PREFACE

Japanese Americans today enter the medical field unfettered by the profound emotional, socioeconomic, and legal obstacles encountered by their predecessors. They are now able to succeed in all aspects of private, academic, and public health care sectors.

This publication, Silent Scars of Healing Hands, provides a unique opportunity for physicians in the Japanese American Medical Association (JAMA) to honor their medical pioneers. By recording the oral histories of as many surviving Japanese American physicians as possible who had served as health care professionals during World War II, it is hoped that the collective glimpse of their early family lives and dynamics, professional training, health care in the incarceration camps, and return to civilian life provides a medical legacy upon which future generations may reflect and appreciate. It is, at the very least, a dramatic kaleidoscope of human emotions and life-changing experiences.

To accomplish this timely project, JAMA was fortunate to have the advice and experience of Lynn Itagaki, Dr. William Sato, Jeannie N. Shinozuka, Dr. Paul I. Terasaki, Dr. James N. Yamazaki, and members of JAMA's Cabinet and Auxiliary Boards. With this insightful help and encouragement, JAMA received a grant on May 15, 2002, from the California Civil Liberties Public Education Program under Program Director Diane Matsuda and State Librarian Dr. Kevin Starr. The selected team that assembled and completed this narrative included consulting anthropologist and oral historian Dr. Gwenn M. Jensen; writer Naomi Hirahara; archival researcher Dr. Louis

Fiset; and our second oral historian, Paul Tsuneishi. Consultants and advisers to the project were Arthur A. Hansen, Director, Center for Oral and Public History at California State University, Fullerton, and Senior Historian, Japanese American National Museum; Irene Y. Hirano, Director of the Japanese American National Museum; and Dr. Don Nakanishi, professor and Director of the UCLA Asian American Studies Center.

Gordon H. Sasaki, MD
President, JAMA (1999–2004)

ACKNOWLEDGMENTS

So many people contributed to the fulfillment of this project. First and foremost, we wish to honor and acknowledge the men and women who participated in our interviews and offered their memories, their photographs, their memorabilia, and their insight. This book is dedicated to their legacy.

Silent Scars of Healing Hands became a reality through the guidance and dream of Dr. Gordon H. Sasaki and the Japanese American Medical Association in conjunction with the Japanese American National Museum and UCLA Asian American Studies Center. Dr. Sasaki and his wife Joanne's persistence in grant-writing and personal underwriting of the project expanded the original concept resulting in twice the number of interviews and doubled the size of the book. We are grateful to Diane Matsuda and the California Civil Liberties Public Education Project for the grant that funded the initial stage of the oral history collection. Dr. Arthur A. Hansen served as project advisor, spearheaded assembling the JAMA team, and coordinated efforts with the Japanese American National Museum and its staff. He and Dr. Sasaki tirelessly nurtured the development of the project. Dr. Don Nakanishi, director of the UCLA Asian American Studies Center, lent his support as project advisor.

JAMA team members included Paul Tsuneishi, who volunteered at the very beginning of the project to help collect oral histories. In addition to conducting some of the interviews he transcribed tapes and provided access to his previous body of interviews especially those of Dr. Clifford Uyeda and Joe Yamakido. Dr. Louis Fiset worked with the JAMA team by providing critical background material and served as project historian. Judy and Mike Soda, of Soda's-Up-The-Creek, Inc., a Del Norte, Colorado, transcription service, completed most of the interview transcriptions.

We are indebted to the following archives, museums, and reference collections for their help and access to their oral history materials and documents: the Japanese American National Museum (Carla Tengan, Maria Kwong, Jamie Henricks, Shawn Iwaoka and others); Pam Macas and the California State University Sacramento, Japanese American Archival Collection; Wayne Maeda, of the Ethnic Studies Department, California State University Sacramento; Karl K. Matsushita and the Japanese American National Library; June Arima Schumann and the Oregon Nikkei Legacy Center; Georgiana White, Special Assistant to the Japanese American Archival Collection for Education and Outreach for California State University Sacramento; and J. K. Yamamoto, *Hokubei Mainichi*, San Francisco.

A number of individuals provided insight and information on the project. Mr. Mamoru Inouye, donated the original cover photo, first published in his 1997 book *The Heart Mountain Story: Photographs by Hansel Mieth and Otto Hagel of the World War II Internment of Japanese Americans*; May Kambara donated papers and memorabilia of her husband, Dr. George K. Kambara; Richard Kinoshita offered direction to military websites and other material; Mary and Eizo Kobayashi gave permission to use their interviews with the late Dr. Yoshiye Togasaki; Barbara Higashi Mosier provided information about her father, Dr. Benjamin Mokoto Higashi; Ron Still, Regimental Historian for the Army Medical Historical Regiment, offered documents on Dr. Kinoshita from the Regiment's collection; and Dennis B. Worthen, Loveland, Ohio, shared his research on Nisei pharmacists.

Dr. Sasaki provided a list of potential narrators, and JAMA team members lent their own contacts and expertise to develop the initial list of interviewees. Through the publication of a press release in a number of venues and an exhibit table at the Tulelake Gathering in September of 2002, many people came forth to offer their assistance. The result was an expanded group of contacts and information. We are most grateful to Jan Kurihara who referred us to Mrs. H. Deki

Seto and Dr. Mac Suzuki, who had been Kurihara's wife's Lil's obstetrician at Tulelake; to Eucaly A. Shirai, for WRA documents on the Tule Lake incident, information on Dr. Hashiba, and for referrals to Dr. Shigeru Hara, Mrs. Yasuka Akamatsu and others; to Fusako Yamamoto, for information on the Togasaki sisters and referrals to their living relatives and friends. (Her husband Masa was drafted before the war in 1941 and, upon his discharge in 1943, went to the University of Chicago Medical School).

Others who provided information about possible narrators were Art Iwasaki, Mae Kakehashi, Col. Jimmie Kanaya, Marian Kanemoto, Margaret Nakano, Yuri Okamoto, Arthur Sato, DDS, Bill Sugiyama, MD, Homer Yasui, MD, and a number of others who stopped by the table at the Tulelake Gathering provided by Lorna Fong, Elaine Chiao and the 2002 Tulelake Committee. Jean Carlson, Sharon Conarton, Cindy Johnson, Karen King, Mike Mackey, Bess Masuda, and Dr. Mary Jane Mosher assisted in various essential ways.

The reissuing of this new volume is due to the efforts of Maria Kwong of JANM, Barry Goy of JAMA, and the staff of Applewood Books. The co-authors are delighted that this material is available to new readers interested in the experience of Japanese Americans during World War II.

The acknowledgments would not be complete without mentioning those who invited Gwenn to stay with them as she conducted interviews in their areas. Thank you to Louis and Joan Fiset, Irving and Jeanne Heller, Raymond and Gloria Heller, Mayumi and Isamu Hirahara, Dee Jensen, Fumi Mochizuki, Mac and Zoe Suzuki, Gus and Teddy Tanaka, and Linda and Dick Van Dyke.

Finally, Gwenn thanks her husband, Jeff Heller, for his continuing support and encouragement, and Naomi credits her husband, Wesley Fukuchi, for providing a clear vision during especially cloudy days.

CONTENTS

INTRODUCTION

Prior to World War II, a premed major was a risky choice for a Nisei (second-generation Japanese American). In spite of being born with all the rights and privileges of U.S. citizenship, the Nisei encountered barriers and hurdles not faced by their European American counterparts. It was toughest on the West Coast, where most Nikkei (people of Japanese heritage) lived; medical schools there generally accepted no more than two students of Asian heritage into entering classes, regardless of their GPAs or other qualifications. Word soon spread that medical schools in the Midwest and East Coast were more receptive, and Nisei found acceptances there. These limitations, born out of prejudice, constrained but did not dissuade Nisei students from pursuing careers in medicine. Despite a litany of legal obstacles and barriers—from alien land laws forbidding property ownership to a ban on citizenship—that circumscribed the lives of their parents, the Issei (the immigrant generation), the Nisei persevered (see, for example, works by the Commission on Wartime Relocation and Internment of Civilians, Roger Daniels, Brian Niiya, and Michi Weglyn, which are listed in "References").

All of this occurred at a time when Nisei with advanced degrees often could not find work in their chosen fields and had to settle for lesser positions or even emigrate to Japan. Once obtained, a medical degree did not guarantee access to the same advantages that European Americans enjoyed. Again, it was different in the Midwest and East, but on the West Coast it was often difficult to find office space or obtain hospital privileges. For that reason, many of the early Issei physicians opened their own clinics and hospitals, particularly in major population centers.

Pearl Harbor changed everything. In the weeks and months after war was declared, Nikkei communities were under siege. Community leaders, including some Issei physicians, were arrested by the FBI and imprisoned in distant Department of Justice internment camps, and the education and fledgling medical careers of Nisei were disrupted.

On February 19, 1942, by order of President Franklin D. Roosevelt, all Nikkei were subject to an indiscriminate and mass incarceration that affected more than 110,000 people. Within weeks, Issei and Nisei doctors found themselves vaccinating long lines of people in anticipation of their imminent removal from homes and businesses. Cast into temporary detention, these same physicians struggled to open clinics and treat patients in facilities ill prepared for the onslaught of families, pregnant women, elderly, and toddlers.

Aware of this historic backdrop of hardship and intolerance, Dr. Gordon Sasaki and the Japanese American Medical Association (JAMA) envisioned a project that would tell the stories of a generation of Nisei physicians who directed health care behind barbed wires. In mid-2002 JAMA obtained funding from a California Civil Liberties Public Education Program project grant that enabled the "Silent Scars of Healing Hands" Oral History Project to begin.

Why oral history? Personal stories are an evocative way to develop the full breadth of historical voices and document significant events. Oral history not only taps into the memories of participants, but it also allows us to elicit answers to questions not considered in the past. Most historical research relies on archival documentary evidence produced contemporaneously, usually by official governmental sources or prominent individuals. Some studies go further and incorporate testimony from personal diaries, letters, or reports by often overlooked participants (see Louis Fiset, Lane Hirabayashi, and Mike Mackey in "References"). Nowhere in War Relocation Authority (WRA) documents, for example, will you read about the need to borrow a carpenter's drill for hip surgery or about etherizing a pig. While Brian Dempster, Arthur Hansen, Naomi Hirahara, Jan Kurahara, Mei Nakano, and Noboru Shirai, to name but a few, have published personal accounts that relate experiences surrounding the World War II detention, no one has focused on the physicians who served the captive communities.

It took forty years after the World War II incarceration before anyone began to study medical practices or health-care workers—and only in the past seventeen years has anything been written on subject. There are a number of unpublished and published articles from students and scholars, including Louis Fiset, Michelle Gutierrez, Pamela Iwasaki, Gwenn Jensen, Troy Kaji, Julie Kikuchi, Susan McKay, Susan Smith, Dennis Worthen, and Fusako Yamamoto. Naomi Hirahara previously conducted interviews and wrote profiles of several medical practitioners for Japanese Community Health, Inc., and other organizations. While just ten people have worked in this area of interest, six continue their pursuit, and three of these—Fiset, Hirahara, and Jensen—were on the JAMA team.

According to a list compiled by Fiset, by World War II there were at least forty-seven Issei and more than fifty Nisei physicians in the United States. It was clear to us from the beginning of this project that all of the Issei physicians were gone, and considering that twenty-five is about the youngest age at which one could hope to become a doctor, any surviving Nisei doctor today would be over eighty. Against high odds, the JAMA team located four doctors who practiced in detention camps, plus one nurse, one health-care worker, and nine individuals who were in the midst of their training and then went on to become physicians. In addition, seven relatives of deceased physicians filled out the story. Doctors were identified and located using the Fiset physician index and through a serendipitous chain of encounters and events. *Silent Scars of Healing Hands* is the result of a year of collecting oral histories and personal memorabilia—Naomi Hirahara, Gwenn Jensen, and Paul Tsuneishi conducted twenty-one interviews in 2002–2003.

This is a book that should have been written thirty years ago when more of the physicians were still alive. Since all of the Issei and many of the Nisei physicians have passed away, *Silent Scars of Healing Hands* is but a glimpse into the lives of a few. The people featured here were in different stages of their medical careers in 1942: they were established physicians, newly minted physicians, premed students, or medical students in training. A number of those interviewed also served in the military, thus shedding light on the experience of Japanese American medical personnel during World War II. *Silent Scars of Healing Hands* proceeds chronologically and gives voice to the experiences of these doctors and health-care workers. In compiling the oral history transcripts into narrative form, we have taken the liberty of editing some of our subjects' dialogue, taking care not to sacrifice content or intent.

In Chapter One, "The Calling," a picture emerges of influential Issei mothers assisting, motivating, and urging their children to pursue medicine in spite of the obstacles they faced. The efforts of these women—a contrast to the image of Japanese women as having no power or influence—defy stereotypic thinking and illustrate that real life is complex.

Chapters Eight and Nine focus on conflicts within the camps which affected the hospital staff peripherally or directly. One incident at Tule Lake involved the beating of Dr. Reece Pedicord, the Chief Medical Officer, a man who engendered the widespread hostility of camp inhabitants as well as the rancor of many on staff. There were other incidents at other camps, notably a walkout of Nikkei hospital physicians and staff at Heart Mountain on June 24, 1943. Although we were able to interview the son of Dr. Robert Kinoshita, who served at the Heart Mountain hospital, Dr. Kinoshita had left prior to the walk-out, and we had no other informants to provide firsthand information. (For an interesting look at that incident, see "The Heart Mountain Hospital Strike of June 24, 1943," by Louis Fiset, in "References.") Other chapters tell the story of how the war affected physicians, their careers, their lives after the war, and their medical practices.

I first became interested in the subject of the World War II mass incarceration while doing research on the relationship between health and stressful and traumatic circumstances. I remembered how I had learned about the incarceration of Japanese Americans quite by accident in the hallways of Los Angeles High School—not in the classroom. Perhaps because I heard about it in an offhand manner,

I was struck by the palpable betrayal, probably more so than if I had learned about it in a more formal setting. I was astounded that such a travesty of justice could be completely unacknowledged by the educational system; I was also surprised that many of the parents of my Sansei (third-generation) classmates did not speak about their experiences with their children.

Later, as I conducted research on the health consequences of the Nikkei incarceration for my dissertation, it was fortuitous that I chose to incorporate oral history as a methodology. After more than fifty interviews, I learned that a resilience rooted in culture was one of the strongest coping mechanisms that protected detainees from stress-induced illness. I also learned that silence became an explicit strategy chosen by many Nisei parents who wanted to protect their children and not have them grow up thinking of them as victims or thinking the worst of our nation.

As I conducted these interviews, I learned that cultural resilience, coupled with doing meaningful work that one loved, could be transformative. Towards the end of the interviewing stage of this project, I began to have reservations about using "Silent Scars of Healing Hands," conceived by the project organizers, as a book title. For one thing, of the eighteen people that I interviewed, few spoke of any "scars" left by their incarceration in America's concentration camps. In fact, doctor after doctor spoke of opportunities to treat patients that neophyte physicians, interns, or med students would not have had on the outside. They described how the hours were long, the patients endless, and the challenges many. The Sakaguchis spoke of losing half their family at Manzanar; Dr. Shigekawa describing her feeling of utter despair at Santa Anita; Richard Kinoshita described how his father developed bleeding ulcers from the sheer stress of treating so many with so few supplies and equipment at Heart Mountain. In spite of these stories, everyone repeatedly emphasized the value of their work. Wounds were not foremost in my mind when I left an interview session.

One by one, each of these interviews ended on such a positive and upbeat note that I left the homes of the interviewees entranced with their lives of triumph and accomplishment. On the surface, certainly, no scars were visible: it was as if everyone had transcended their experience of incarceration and transformed themselves into dynamic, charming people.

It was only later, in the quiet of my office, as I reviewed the transcripts without their indomitable presence to distract me, that the scars borne by these remarkable people became perceptible. You will read about these scars in the coming chapters. Finally, I saw that the book's title was even more appropriate.

It is important to have a passion in life. In the pages that follow, you will meet many men and women who embody a passion for medicine, and because of this passion, they made—and continue to make—a difference in people's lives.

Gwenn M. Jensen, PhD
August 2003

SILENT SCARS OF HEALING HANDS

1. THE CALLING

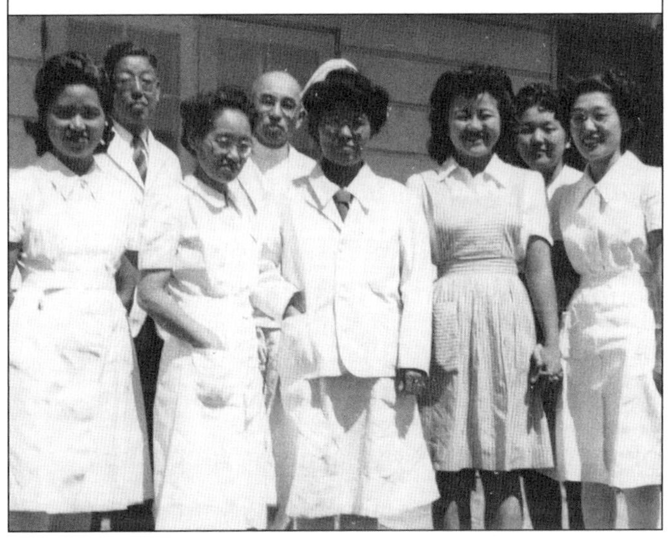

So she said, "Go into medicine, and it will be good for you."

—Shigeru Hara, MD, regarding his mother's advice in 1929

Japanese immigrants first entered Hawai'i, then a territory of the United States, en masse in 1868 to work on sugar plantations. California and other western states subsequently recruited the Issei, or first-generation Japanese Americans, as farm workers to grow and harvest fruits and vegetables. These early pioneers were primarily bachelors, and the U.S. sought to limit the number of these laborers allowed into the country through the Gentlemen's Agreement of 1908. However, a loophole in the agreement led to an unintended result: the immigration of picture brides. Now Japanese Americans were establishing themselves as families, and medical services were needed more than ever.

MASAKO (KUSAYANAGI) MIURA

Masako (Kusayanagi) Miura was born on June 29, 1914, in Pasadena, California, to Japanese immigrants. A year later, her family moved to downtown Los Angeles in the back of her father Takejiro's store, Pacific Trading Company. Miura had been a "rather sickly child." "I think I got every infectious disease practically. I had measles three times, but no chicken pox. I had mumps, and I think that's about it," she said. A number of Nikkei (people of Japanese heritage) doctors in Los Angeles, including Dr. Paul K. Ito, a first-generation Japanese American, or Issei, pediatrician born in 1888 and trained at Loma Linda University in Southern California, provided aid to children suffering from such ailments. At the time many early Issei physicians, educated in Japan, practiced on the West Coast. They were required, however, to pass an English-language examination to attain their medical licenses.

When Miura was five, she was badly burned at her aunt's house. "I had on a flannel dress. Of course, in those days, they didn't have any fireplace, they just had gas heaters. So I backed up on it, and my dress caught on fire and I got burned. So I remember having them put black tarry stuff on my legs. I had to [lay] on my stomach for quite a long time until they healed." While her parents worked, she had to lie on the counter in the back of her father's store. Sympathetic salesmen offered her dimes and nickels. "I used to put it in my piggy bank. I accumulated quite a bit at that time," she laughed.

After graduating from Hollywood High School in 1931, Miura went to Japan with her family to spend a year with her ailing grandfather. In Tokyo, she encountered some disfigured people who were sitting and begging on the street. They were lepers. "I thought, 'I'd like to do something to help them out.'" It was then Miura decided to become a physician.

While in Japan for a year in the early 1930s, Miura attended the Kaisen Girl's School in Setagaya, an area within Tokyo. At one point, her father told her, "You don't have to go to school because girls get married anyway."

"Well," Miura replied, "if you don't send me to school, that's all right. I'll get a job."

Seeing his daughter's determination, Takejiro relented. In 1932, Miura entered the University of Southern California (USC), where she was active in the International Relations Club and Amazons, a women's service organization now called Helen of Troy. She pursued her dream with a major in premed.

WILLIAM SATO

In the case of William Sato, his path to become a medical doctor was influenced by his father's sense of philanthropy. His father, Yoriyuki, a former farmer, had established a flower shop in South Pasadena on Fair Oaks Avenue in the 1920s. From their profits, his mother, Makako, had carefully saved five thousand dollars, a small fortune in those days, for the education of her children. But to her dismay, her savings would be used for another cause entirely.

In 1928, the Japanese community in Southern California celebrated a large legal victory.

In 1926, Dr. Kikuo Tashiro, a Nagasaki-born physician, and four other Issei doctors decided to build a modern hospital for the Japanese community. Up till then, there had been only small clinics and a small hospital at Turner and Amelia streets in Los Angeles' Little Tokyo district had been expanded after the 1918 influenza epidemic. The expansion was prompted after infected Japanese Americans were turned away from hospitals operated by and for the white community.

Yoriyuki had once been admitted to the limited Turner Street hospital for an appendectomy. "He had a bad time of it after the operation," Sato explained. "I remember that was first time I ever saw my father cry because of the pain."

The California Secretary of State refused to let the physicians incorporate to raise funds for the hospital. In turn, the physicians sued in 1927, and the case went to the US Supreme Court in 1928. The court determined that the physicians could not be barred from incorporating to build a hospital, even in light of U.S.–Japan Treaty agreements or state alien land laws. Among other things, these treaty agreements provided for limited Japanese immigration to the United States and the alien land laws barred non-citizens, specifically Asian immigrants who were not allowed to become citizens until 1952, from owning property.

Led by the "Big Five" Issei doctors (Kikuo Tashiro, Daishiro Kuroiwa, Fusataro Nakaya, Toru Ozasa, and Matsuta Takahashi), a fund-raising campaign was launched throughout the Japanese American community. As a result, Yoriyuki donated his children's college fund to the effort. "My mother was so mad," remembered Sato. "I don't think she ever forgave him."

Even during the depths of the Great Depression, the community raised more than $129,000. A lot on East First and Fickett streets in Boyle Heights, a community just east of Little Tokyo, was purchased under the name of a young Stanford-educated Nisei physician George Yogoro Takeyama. In December 1929, a 42-bed Japanese Hospital was inaugurated, complete with three operating rooms, an X-ray room, and laboratory.

Even though his mother Makako lost her children's education fund, she decided that the establishment of the hospital would serve as an important personal legacy for her children. "She encouraged us to go into medicine one way or another," said Sato. And indeed, Sato and his younger brother, George, did become doctors, while his sister, Jane, went on to become a nurse.

SAKAYE SHIGEKAWA

Sakaye Shigekawa was born a twin to Issei parents in South Pasadena on January 6, 1913. Her father was a gardener and a part owner of a Long Beach hog farm, and her mother was owner of a grocery store. When Shigekawa was a teenager, her father had double pneumonia, which developed into empyema, an infection in the lung cavity, requiring him to be hospitalized for almost six months. "In those days there were no antibiotics. You had to depend on your own immune system to carry you through, and, of course, oxygen and all the other, like drainage of the empyema and so on, but no medication whatsoever. I was at the hospital to see my father everyday. At first he was in the Japanese Hospital... But the facilities there couldn't take care of him completely, so he was moved to the Good Samaritan Hospital.

"I took the streetcar and would go to the Good Samaritan Hospital, which is located on Seventh or Sixth and Wilshire. I got acquainted with all the nurses and his private nurse, and the doctor was very kind. I thought I'd like to be what he is doing for my father. So that was the beginning of my feeling for wanting to study medicine.

"However, I knew I wasn't that smart, but my mother said, 'Well, if another human being can do this certain [thing], you're another human being, so if you try hard enough, you should be able to do it.

"So in spite of the fact that I wasn't too much of a scholar, and I wasn't too interested in school, I had to work hard to get where I am, because [my] one purpose in my life was to study medicine. I wanted to be a doctor."

SHIGERU HARA

If Shigeru Hara had not contracted tuberculosis during his senior year in high school in Sacramento, he might have never considered medicine. Born on September 16, 1911, Hara was raised on a farm in Sacramento Valley. When he was twelve, his father started a garage business. "So we grew up working with cars in the early days," said Hara.

In 1929, Hara developed tubercular peritonitis, a tuberculosis of the abdominal cavity. To address the intestinal obstruction caused by this condition, Hara had surgery in February 1929. A second surgery followed in April 1930.

"At that time they had no treatment except food, rest, and sun baths. I went through it all. It kept me at home for about two or three years," said Hara. He had to drop out of his 1929 graduating class; he finally graduated from high school in 1932.

"Because of that, my mother used to tell me, 'You're not going to be too strong, you know. You might as well take something that you don't have to work too hard [physically].'

"We had a general practice doctor in our building, renting from us. And she said, 'Look, he charges three dollars, just to see a patient. Go into medicine, and it will be good for you.'"

MARY (SAKAGUCHI) ODA

As with many of the other Nisei interviewed, Mary (Sakaguchi) Oda's mother Hisaji often gave her children career advice. "She was always telling my brother Sanbo to become a doctor. She was always telling my two older brothers to become dentists," Oda said.

By the time Oda was three years old, her family had moved to rural North Hollywood. Her parents had a total of seven children.

One day Oda's mother sat down with three of her children: Chibo, 17; Mary, 13; and Lily, 12. "She looked at Lily's hands and didn't say a word. She looked at my hands and didn't say a word. She looked at Chibo's, and she said, 'Chibo, you have good hands. You should be a dentist.'

"So I said, 'Mama, what are you looking at?'

"So she said, 'You can tell how good a person's hand is by the number of central whorls on the fingertips.'"

Chibo had seven whorls, and Mary had six. "My mother didn't tell me to be a dentist. She just didn't say anything. She just said, 'Don't be a teacher.'"

BENJAMIN MASAYOSHI TANAKA

As his son Augustus "Gus" Masashi Tanaka tells it, Benjamin Tanaka was a young man with an independent streak. Born in Rappahoihoi on the eastern coast of the island of Hawai'i, Tanaka did not know whether his birth year was 1881 or 1882 since the government did not always bother to register the births of children of plantation workers. At the age of either eleven or twelve, Tanaka stowed away on a boat headed for Seattle, Washington, never to see his parents again.

Eventually traveling east into the interior of Washington, Tanaka worked as a school boy in Sandpoint, Idaho, near Coeur d'Alene. "His dream was after graduation from high school [was to] become an engineer," said his son Gus. "Well, he got one whale of a tummy ache one night, and he got progressively ill. People wanted him to go to the hospital, but of course [being] alone—there was no such thing as insurance—he had no one to help him financially, and he certainly didn't have any money.

"When he got too sick to resist, some people took him to the hospital and a diagnosis of a ruptured appendix was made on him. The doctor insisted he had to be operated on or he was going to die. Dad said he got up off the examining table to go home to get ready to die, because there was no way he could finance it.

"He said that this doctor sat down and had a good, long talk with him, and said that he would not charge him. In fact, he would pay off the hospital bill for him if he would promise to be just as kind to some unfortunate guy himself when he got older and more mature and could afford to do those things.

"At that point, he considered how wonderful the profession of medicine was. He changed his mind about wanting to go to an engineering school and decided he was going to go into medicine."

But as a "runway kid" with "no money, no family, no help," where would he attend college? "He looked around and wrote to a number of schools and found that the cheapest place where he could go to undergraduate school was the University of North Dakota," said Gus. There he befriended a Chinese American from Hawai'i, Min Hin Lee, and together the two former Islanders supported each other financially. They took turns attending classes and working. They finally graduated six years later than their entrance class.

TOGASAKI SISTERS

The Togasaki home in San Francisco was a lively, stimulating place. The patriarch, Kikumatsu, had come to the United States to study law but became involved in an art store business and eventually an import-export enterprise. His wife Shige, a devout Christian and descendant of a founder of the Japan Women's Christian Temperance Union, assisted picture brides in adjusting to their new lives in the United States.

"She would be helping families," explained Shinobu, the youngest son of Kikumatsu and his second wife Sugi. "They'd say, 'Well, who's taking care of your family?'

"And she'd say, 'Kazue.' And Kazue was."

Kazue was the couple's oldest daughter. The oldest child and son

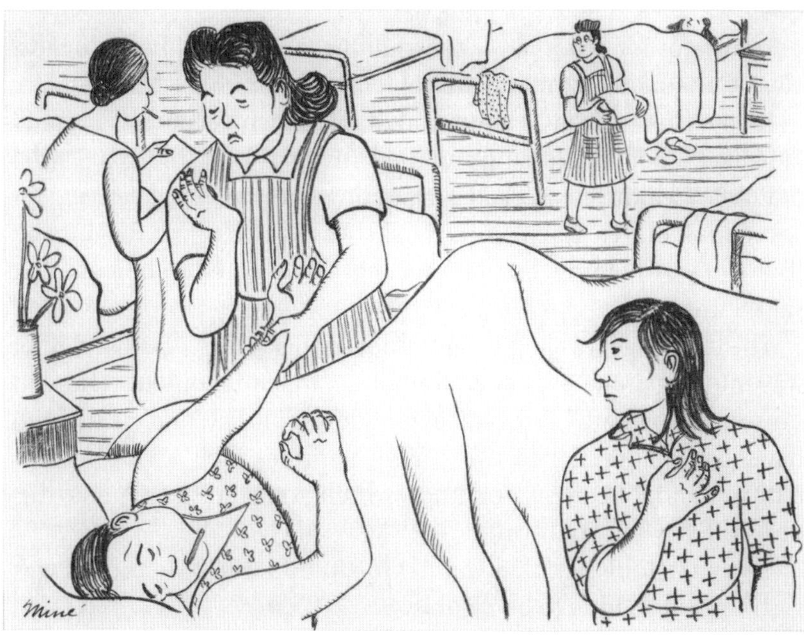

An illustration of a hospital scene at Topaz by artist Miné Okubo.

was Kiyoshi, followed by Kazue, then another son Susumu, and five other daughters—Mitsuye, Yoshiye, Chiye, Teru, and Yaye. (After Shige died from food poisoning, Kikumatsu married Sugi Hida, who gave birth to his ninth child, Shinobu.) All six daughters eventually went into medicine as either doctors or nurses.

When the 1906 earthquake hit San Francisco, Kikumatsu's art store was in ruins, but the family was still thinking of public service. They converted a Japanese American church into a makeshift hospital and assisted injured individuals as much as they could.

Often sent by her mother to help immigrant families, these activities apparently had an impact on Kazue. "She told me one incident where she vividly remembered that a child was choking on mucus in the nose, and the mother right in front of her just virtually put her mouth over [the nose] and sucked everything out. That's how that child survived. That gave her such a strong impression, she said that that's one of the turning points in her life," commented Kazue's nephew Gordon Togasaki. During this time, young Kazue also served as translator for a woman who would become one of her role models, a Canadian doctor and ardent feminist.

Kazue first trained as a nurse at Stanford University's Children's Hospital School of Nursing and the University of California School of Public Health. She worked as a public health nurse but yearned for something more. "Kazue thought she was smarter than the doctors that she was helping. So she said that she wanted to be a doctor," said Shinobu.

The challenge was to get the support of her father. "Dad at dinner was interrogation," explained Shinobu. "I mean, not like, 'Did you do something bad?' But intellectual development, and he liked to have all his children there every night at dinner. Well, Kazue became a nurse, and, of course, you know, when you study as a nurse, dinner shift is when you work....

"Later she told me, 'Dad wanted me to be a doctor because I was getting paid so little to be a nurse.'

"I said, 'I don't believe you.... Dad wanted you to be a doctor because he didn't like you missing dinner. That was the biggest reason.'

"She said, 'Oh, you're absolutely right.'"

Kazue became the first Japanese American student to be accepted at the Women's Medical College of Pennsylvania. Following in her footsteps as future doctors were her younger sisters, Yoshiye and Teru.

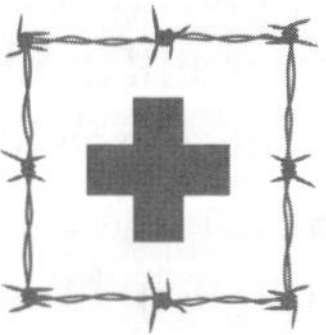

2. PREWAR MEDICAL TRAINING AND PRACTICES

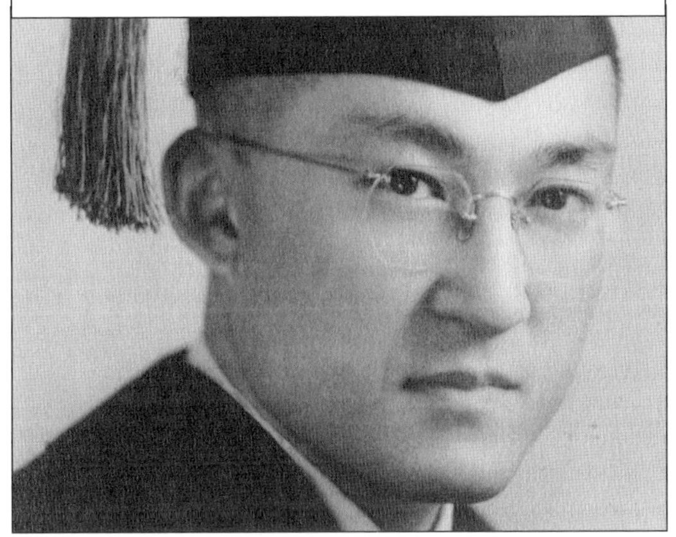

"Because of what those damned Japs are doing in Manchuria, you will never get a job."

—Mary Sakaguchi Oda, MD, relating what a professor said to her at UCLA

SHIGERU HARA
SANBO SAKAGUCHI
MASAHARU RICHARD SETO
HENRY IWAO SUGIYAMA
JAMES N. YAMAZAKI

In the 1930s, medical school applicants were not required to have undergraduate degrees. "In those days, they only required three years, junior year, to get into medical school. You didn't have to have a B.A. or a B.S.," explained Shigeru Hara. He went to Sacramento City Junior College for two years before transferring to the University of California at Berkeley. After a year, he and a fellow classmate Henry Sugiyama, affectionately called "Sugi," looked for medical schools to apply to. "... he and I both applied to the University of California Medical School, and we both got turned down. His grades were better than mine, but you know, they didn't like the Japanese too well in those days."

Although many Nisei physicians spoke of racial and gender quotas in the selection of medical students during the prewar era, admission policies regarding minorities and women were not openly advertised. Nisei actually did attend the University of California Medical School, but in limited numbers. At the time, there was only one medical school in the UC system and it was located in San Francisco. Among the licensed Japanese American physicians incarcerated during World War II, only five had graduated from the University of California Medical School before 1934 as found by Fiset. Although some were accepted by Loma Linda University (a Seventh Day Adventist school), Stanford University, and the University of Oregon, many Nisei medical students headed east.

Born in San Francisco on September 4, 1912, Masaharu Richard Seto had been raised in Sacramento. His mother had joined the American Red Cross during World War I, making bandages out of white bed sheets. He completed his undergraduate education at the University of Minnesota, paying for his tuition from money made working on farms during the summer, in addition to jobs for the Works Progress Administration (WPA) and as a houseboy. The University of Minnesota had a policy against accepting Californians

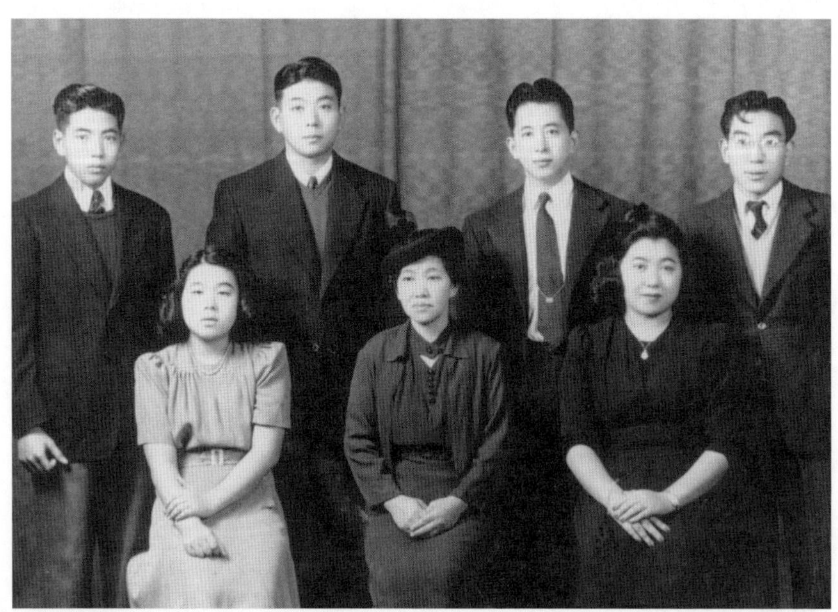

ABOVE: Seto family portrait, October 1939, Sacramento. Standing, L to R: Louie (1925–1993), Haruo (Hilo) (1914–2000), Masa (1912–1985), and Joe (1919–1987). Seated L to R: Dorothy (b. 1936), Uta Seto (1891–1987), and Annie (1926–1991). BELOW: Masaharu Richard Seto's medical doctorate diploma, granted June 11, 1941.

Senatus
Universitatis Marquettensis
Omnibus Has Litteras Visuris
Salutem in Domino

Nos Rector et Senatus ex commendatione Decani Professorumque Collegii Nostri certiores facimus omnes dilectum nobis alumnum

Masaharu Richard Seto, A.B.

periculo facto ad Medicinae Doctoris gradum in solemni Senatus nostri Sessione fuisse provectum, cumque singulis juribus et privilegiis ad istum gradum pertinentibus a Nobis fuisse donatum. In cujus rei testimonium, Nos ad id muneris publica auctoritate delegati praesentes litteras manu nostra subscriptas et Universitatis sigillo munitas dedimus. Milwaukiae in Statu Wisconsinensi die undecima Junii Anno Domini MCMXLI

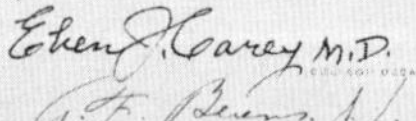

to its medical school, so Seto looked to the next best thing: Marquette University in Milwaukee, Wisconsin.

While getting his medical degree from Marquette, his father died. His brother Hilo stepped in and supported the family while Seto was at medical school. To supplement his income from other jobs, Seto also manned the bar for parties held by a fraternity and acquired the moniker, "Masa the Bartender," according to his wife Hideko "Deki" Nakazawa Seto.

Seto told other Sacramento Nisei about Marquette, including Shigeru Hara and Henry Sugiyama. For two years after completing his premed studies at UC Berkeley, Sugiyama was doing anything he could to raise money for his advanced education. "I worked in a liquor store. I worked in a grocery store. I worked out on a farm. I picked fruit.... I decided I still wanted to go into medicine, so I applied to the east," said Sugiyama, "Just like that I got into medical school."

So Sugiyama and Hara prepared to follow Masaharu Seto, who was a class above them at Marquette. There was only one catch: Marquette was a Jesuit school and Sugiyama was Buddhist. "I had to promise that whenever they had to go to mass on Friday that I wouldn't study for two hours," said Sugiyama.

In 1939, the Northern Californians were joined by a Southern Californian, James N. Yamazaki, the son of Los Angeles Episcopal minister John Misao Yamazaki; Sanbo Sakaguchi, a former UCLA classmate of James Yamazaki; and Kinji Hara, younger brother of Shigeru Hara, followed in 1941.

ROBERT S. KINOSHITA

Like the older Benjamin Masayoshi Tanaka, Robert S. Kinoshita, the son of successful furniture manufacturers and real estate investors, was born in the Territory of Hawai'i, but unlike Tanaka, had proper papers recording his date and place of birth. "... My Dad had both Japanese and United States citizenship," explained Kinoshita's son Richard. "But when you reach the age of majority in Hawai'i, the United States government required you to choose one or the other. They would not let you have both."

At McKinley High School on the Island of O'ahu, Kinoshita had entered the U.S. Army ROTC program. "... In order to become a United States Army officer, you have to be a citizen. So he chose United States citizenship." Kinoshita, whose mother's health had had suffered in Hawai'i's tropical heat, also wanted him to become a doctor. But to attain this goal, he would have to go either to Japan or to the mainland. The University of Hawai'i had a cooperative program with the University of Nebraska, so after spending a year at the former institution, he traveled to the Midwest. By 1929, he had not only obtained his bachelor's degree from the University of Nebraska, but also had received his commission as a second lieutenant in the Army Reserve infantry. He went on to medical school at his alma mater and upon his graduation in 1934, traveled to Portland, Oregon, where he filled an internship at Emanuel Hospital vacated by an injured friend. There he met an European American nursing student, Evelyn. They made plans to get married but were hindered by Oregon's anti-miscegenation laws. "The state of Oregon would not issue interracial marriage licenses," explained Richard. "They had to go to another state [Washington] to be married."

In 1936, during the Depression, Dr. Kinoshita became a medical-surgical consultant of the Southern Oregon district of the Civilian Conservation Corps (CCC). "The Civilian Conservation Corps was a program set up by [President] Roosevelt to employ young men," explained Richard. "The idea was that they would get a job. They would do work in the forests or wherever the work needed to be done. Three-quarters of their salary would go back to their families to help them, and, of course, they got to keep the rest, which wasn't very much. Dad thought that was a pretty good idea [to work there], because it was going to be hard to open your own practice during those hard times."

Kinoshita was assigned to the Medford District, which comprised seventy thousand square miles in both Oregon and California. Approximately one hundred Army Reserve officers were assigned to this district, as the CCC program was administered by the army. Within this vast area, the Kinoshitas moved a number of times. "The district surgeon, when my father started the job, gave him one order.

And that was that if my father felt capable of anything that he had to do, that he was to go ahead and do it, because this was a rural area. There was no time to have a conference about it. There wasn't a lot of telephones or radios. If you were going to have an emergency, you were going to have to do it, unless you didn't feel qualified. That was another thing, my father never felt unqualified on anything, I don't think." In time, Kinoshita was elevated to district surgeon, responsible for forty-four camps.

MASAMICHI "MAC" SUZUKI

Born in Acampo, California, a small town between Sacramento and Stockton, Masamichi "Mac" Suzuki entered the University of California Medical School in 1939 after graduating Phi Beta Kappa from the University of California at Berkeley. A record 10 percent of the class were of Asian heritage, including his friend Edwin Nishimura. Suzuki and Nishimura together worked on a research project to create a parabiotic rat–artificial Siamese twins–and then answer the question: After suturing two rats together and allowing them to heal, do the blood vessels unite or do they remain separate?

They used sodium pentathol as their anesthesia and silk thread for suturing. Instead of a sterilizer, all the instruments were placed in Lysol. "Then the next thing, we've got to remove the hair," said Suzuki. "We found there was a depilatory powder which, when applied, will remove the hair. You leave it on for a little while, just scrape off the hair, resulting in nice clean skin to work on. After anesthetizing the pair, we made our incision from the shoulder down into the abdomen and opened up the peritoneal cavity, sewed together the scapula, and united the abdominal cavities."

Suzuki and Nishimura created two pair of parabiotic rats. "Now we had to prove whether the blood vessels were uniting or not, our main study."

Through special arrangements with the radiation laboratory, the two students injected radioactive sodium chloride into a jugular vein of one parabiotic rat, while removing a small amount of blood from the other. A Geiger counter determined how quickly the sodium solution was transmitted. And sure enough, within a few minutes the blood showed the radioactivity.

"We said, 'The blood vessels must combine.'

"Well, the question came up, could radioactive sodium move by way of the peritoneal cavity, since we united the peritoneal cavity, could it spread to the other rat, and get back into the bloodstream. That was the argument Professor Simpson brought up. At the end of the year, students had to make a presentation. Ed and I flipped a coin. If I recall, I won. I presented the paper, and I thought I did real well.

"Professor Simpson said, 'Well, you know that doesn't prove it. It's possible that the sodium solution from the peritoneal cavity could have gone across to the other and reabsorbed.' Fortunately our paper was the last for the morning. At lunchtime we decided to kill our pretty little Siamese twin, which was the cutest thing; running together all over the place.... We finally killed it, and then washed the blood out and injected India ink. Sure enough the visible blood vessels filled with ink crossed to the other side immediately. We returned that afternoon to show the results to the professors. I think that's the reason why Ed and I got an 'A' in anatomy."

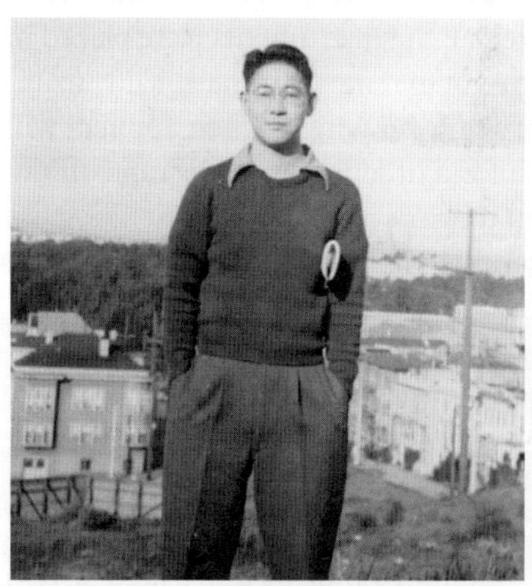

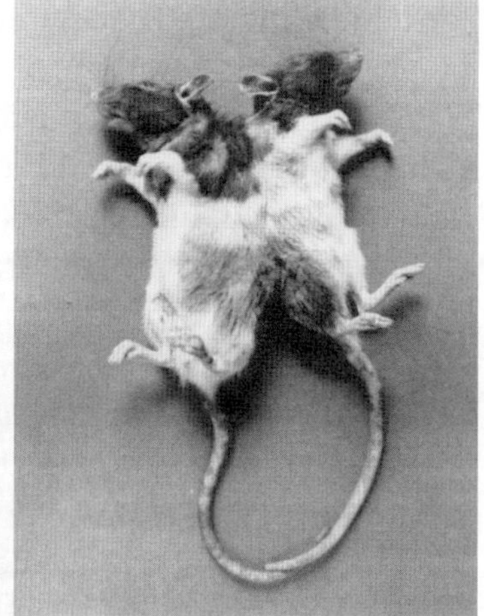

Medical student Edwin Nishimura (left) and (right)
Nishimura and Mac Suzuki's parabiotic rat.

Y. FRED FUJIKAWA

Like other Nisei aspiring doctors, Yasuhiko Fred Fujikawa, who was attending Creighton Medical School in Nebraska, spent his summers selling fruits and vegetables to earn money for his tuition. Born in 1910, he would return to his home in Los Angeles on his breaks to work twelve-to-fourteen-hour days for Three Star Produce Market. Little did he know that this work would result in valuable contacts for his medical internship.

"One summer I was working in Glendale," said Fujikawa, "and one of my customers was a doctor, F. T. Reid. He took an interest in me because I was a medical student and I had finished [in] three years. He asked me one day where I was going to intern, and I told him that I would certainly like to intern at the big general [Los Angeles County General Hospital], but they had never taken a Japanese American.

"He said, 'Oh, is that so? Let me see what I can find out.' He was a very close friend of Roger Jessup of the L.A. County Board of Supervisors. He was superintendent of charities, I think he was. About a couple of a weeks later he came by and he said, 'Fred, I'll tell you what you do. You buy a box of a certain brand of cigars; go make an appointment to see Roger Jessup.' Which I did.... I took my cigars and I went up there and Roger Jessup greeted me like an old friend, you know. Shook my hand, and told me not to worry."

Fujikawa did indeed get the internship in 1934, and like the other interns, received no pay. Instead, they received uniforms, laundry service, and room and board on the hospital grounds. Another Japanese American intern at the facility was Dr. Megumi Shinoda, who, along with Kazue Togasaki, became the first women of Japanese ancestry to receive medical degrees in 1933.

The internships consisted of fifteen to twenty services, including surgery, neuromedicine, orthopedic surgery, pediatrics, radiology, and psychiatry. Each service took six weeks to complete. "We didn't have any eight-hour shifts," said Fujikawa. "We worked until we were through."

In the mid-1930s, medical technology and treatments were limited. "In the old days, we had to use our senses: eyes, ears, and hands more, and we had to use more judgment than I think they do now," said Fujikawa.

"There is an old story that goes around," he explained. "This doctor walked into the ward and he sniffed, and he said, 'There's typhoid in here.' ... And I remember another doctor at a conference one time who looked at a chest X-ray and he said, 'This is silicosis.' And some doctor asked him, 'How do you know for sure?' 'You can smell it,' he said–on an X-ray. Actually he was a very experienced doctor from a mining area in Missouri."

After his two-year internship, twenty-six-year-old Fujikawa opened his own medical office in August 1936 in the Japanese American fishing colony of Terminal Island, where his father was working in a cannery. The opening of his office at 194 Cannery Street was celebrated at a local "China-meshi" or Chinese-style, restaurant. Fujikawa was not the only doctor on the island. There were also Dr. S. Okami at 190½ Terminal Way and Dr. M. Kimura at 707½ Tuna Street, as well as two dentists.

The medical practice was a one-man operation. "I didn't even have a nurse.... I used to do circumcisions and tonsillectomies and drainage of abscesses, and many procedures right in the office by myself." Many times, Fujikawa would not charge his patients—even those who woke him up at two o'clock in the morning—because he had been used to working for no wages during his internship years. "Then when I went into practice, I couldn't charge those patients... Something I'd been doing for nothing all those years. That's the reason why sometimes I'd say, 'Ah, that's all right.'"

But his patients insisted that they pay something. Often it would be one dollar.

MARY (SAKAGUCHI) ODA

As she had decided early on as a teenager, Mary (Sakaguchi) Oda majored in bacteriology with hopes of working in a research laboratory. But during her second year as an undergraduate at the University of California at Los Angeles (UCLA) in the late 1930s, she met with one of her professors, Dr. Beckwith, for her annual review. "You're doing well," he told her. "What are you going to do with your major?"

"I just want to work in a lab," she told him. "I want to be a bacteriologist."

"If I were you, I would quit."

"Why, Dr. Beckwith?"

"Because of what those damned Japs are doing in Manchuria, you will never get a job."

In those days, no one said "damn publicly," explained Oda. The epic film on the Civil War, *Gone with the Wind*, had made its debut around that time, and Rhett Butler's concluding line to heroine Scarlett O'Hara, "Frankly I don't give a damn," had created a sensation. Upon hearing "Jap," Oda thought, "I'm not one of those. I was born here, I'm an American." Interestingly enough, Oda was more shocked by her professor's use of "damn" than "Jap."

Oda then went to the associate professor of bacteriology, Miriam Green. "Is that true, that if I graduate in bacteriology, I'll never have a job?"

Dr. Green didn't hesitate in answering. "Yes," she said.

"What should I do? I'm majoring in bacteriology."

"Go into nursing; you'll always have a job. If you're a nurse, you'll always have a job."

Oda then went home and spoke to her mother. She said nothing about her professor's comment about "those damned Japs in Manchuria."

"Mama," Oda said, "the professor says that if I major in bacteriology, I'll never have a job and she told me to be a nurse."

Oda's mother Hisaji adamantly rejected that idea. Hisaji revealed that her older sister had been a nurse and that she had died in the 1918 flu epidemic in Japan. "My sister worked so hard and did such dirty work," her mother said. "I don't want you to do work that dirty, that hard…."

Up to this time, Oda's mother had supported her brother's path to become a doctor, but had not said much to Oda herself.

"Mama, can I be a doctor?" Oda finally asked.

Her mother agreed, and in 1941, she was one out of three Japanese Americans and eleven women accepted to the University of California's only medical school, located in San Francisco. Apparently, the school had anticipated that many of the young men would go off to war, so women would be able to fill that gap. Renting a room in Berkeley, Oda joined the two Nisei—Yosh Morita and Jerry Ikawa—in medical studies and proceeded to have the best several months of her life.

SAKAYE SHIGEKAWA

Even though her USC physiology professor made a comment that it was too difficult to get into medical school, Sakaye Shigekawa apparently didn't pay any attention. In terms of women, USC medical school had eventually accepted two women, including a USC graduate, Masako (Kusayanagi) Miura, and Tsutayo Ichioka. But it was 1937 and everyone believed that there were quotas limiting the number of women and minorities, such as Japanese Americans. Upon the recommendation of another USC classmate, Shigekawa applied to Stritch Loyola Medical School in Chicago and was accepted. Her mother's grocery store business helped fund her education.

Shigekawa was suddenly among people who had never seen a person of Asian descent before. "I think they were more curious about my reaction to things," she said about her male classmates. "So they would pull all kinds of tricks on me, but not to hurt me." At times male anatomical parts from a cadaver would land up on her desk. Another time it was a condom.

Describing herself as "rather naive" and "pretty sheltered," Shigekawa would hold up the items and ask, "Oh, what's this? Who put it here?"

Everyone laughed in response and Shigekawa said to herself, "Gee, what's so funny about that?"

One time a professor seemed to single her out in class with his relentless questions. "I got really upset. At the end of the lecture, he came up to me and he said, 'Well, you know I wasn't picking on you actually, I was just teasing you because everybody else was teasing you.'

"I just shrugged my shoulders and walked away. So that happened, but I didn't let it bother me too much, I just ignored the professor after that.... I just thought, 'Consider the source.' But that's the way

I felt whenever things like that would happen. I didn't make a big thing of it. I just felt I was glad to be there, and I mean I was glad to be able to study medicine."

KATSUMI JAMES NAKADATE

Katsumi James Nakadate, a Nisei born in Portland on February 3, 1914, did so well at Willamette University in Salem, Oregon, that he was easily accepted to the University of Oregon Medical School after three years of undergraduate work. He was not the only Asian: his entering class in 1935 had a total of five students of Asian descent.

"As far as I'm concerned, I didn't have any discrimination," explained Nakadate. "The only discrimination that I could think of was I could not get an internship on the West Coast.... I applied two or three places. I won't even say where they were.... But when I went back east quick like, I could have gone to three or four different places: three of them in Chicago and a couple in New York. But I went to Indiana, a little place in Indiana. They called it St. Catherine's; it's a Catholic institution where I took my internship. So I became a Catholic."

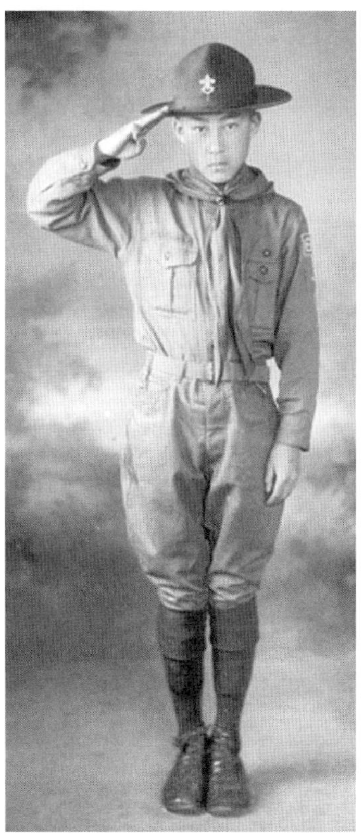

Dr. Katsumi J. Nakadate in Boy Scout uniform, Portland, Oregon, 1927, at thirteen years of age.

Nakadate, who became an Eagle Scout with the Boy Scouts at age fourteen while he grew up in Portland, had stayed close to the organization even through his medical training and internship. While at the University of Oregon Medical School in Portland, he was a Scout Master, leading twenty-one young Japanese Americans in

Troop 123. Completely devoted to Scouting and its "Be Prepared" motto, Nakadate said, "I felt that the younger fellows should be Americans, one hundred percent Americans, as it were." It was his connection to the Boy Scouts that would help Nakadate in a tangible way after the bombing of Pearl Harbor.

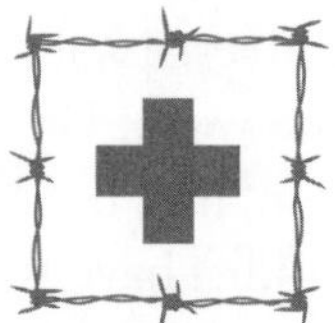

3. PEARL HARBOR

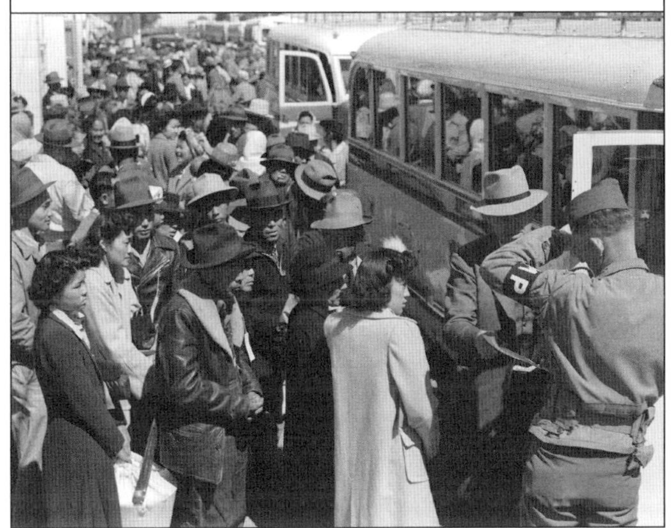

I remember Sugi wrote a prescription for one patient, and that patient promptly dumped it down the toilet, because he didn't trust a Japanese doctor.

—Shigeru Hara, MD, regarding an incident involving Henry Iwao Sugiyama, his friend and fellow resident

MASAMICHI “MAC” SUZUKI

Mac Suzuki was in his third year of medical school at the University of California, located in San Francisco, in the early winter of 1941. On Sunday morning, December 7, 1941, “I happened to be sitting outside on the back porch,” remembered Suzuki. “Many homes in San Francisco had a narrow, long backyard. I heard someone shouting, ‘the Japs have attacked Pearl Harbor!’”

“So I ran inside and turned the radio on, and sure enough, Pearl Harbor was being attacked. But the interesting fact, I was working at the Laguna Honda Home for old sick patients during the Christmas vacation. I first worked as an orderly, then switched to [being] the telephone switch board operator... Whenever [a] blackout occurred, my duty was to inform the engineers and the superintendent. The police department would call all the hospitals before the actual blackout so the engineer could turn on the emergency electric generator.

“The first time when the blackout occurred, we didn’t receive the call early enough. Doctors were performing an emergency gallbladder operation with several flashlights and the surgeon completed the operation.”

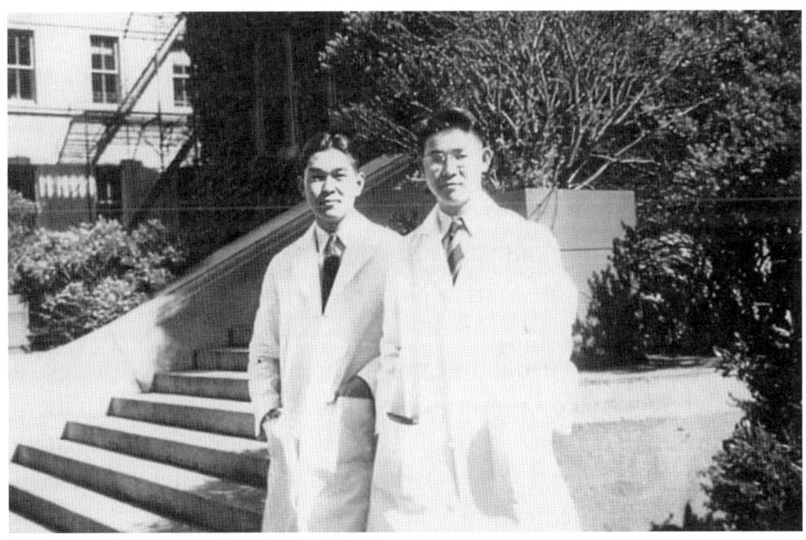

Edwin Nishimura, left, and Mac Suzuki, right, at University of California Medical School, San Francisco.

Suzuki was working the switchboard that evening. "You couldn't see anything at all. The red lights were flashing all over the switchboard," he said. "Finally, some friend came to my rescue with a flashlight; we were able to straighten it out."

These blackouts happened often. "Announcers would say over the radio that an unidentified plane is approaching Golden Gate followed by blackout. Then later, it would be announced that the flight was friendly, we could turn our lights back on. The shades [were] down and blacked out from the outside. There was no light. We used to study in the closet."

SHIGERU HARA & HENRY IWAO SUGIYAMA

Both Dr. Shigeru Hara and Dr. Henry Sugiyama, recent graduates from Marquette Medical School, had internships at Sacramento County Hospital. They lived at the hospital and were paid $35 a month for their work. The Eli Lilly Company, a drug company, had given each of them a small medical bag with a percussion hammer, stethoscope, and a flashlight.

"One day the supervisor called us and said, 'You know they've been at war, Japan attacked Pearl Harbor.' We had never heard of Pearl Harbor," remembered Hara. The supervisor told them, "There may be some kind of incident here and there, so be careful."

According to Sugiyama, "then they took my flashlight away because they said I was going to get up on the roof of the hospital and signal the Zeroes [Japanese war planes]." His father, in fact, had been picked up by the FBI and later placed in alien internment camps in Missoula, Montana; Bismarck, North Dakota; and finally Santa Fe, New Mexico.

Work resumed as usual, but not without unsettling episodes. "I remember Sugi wrote a prescription for one patient, and that patient promptly dumped it down the toilet, because he didn't trust a Japanese doctor," recalled Hara. Later, someone else wrote the man a prescription for the same medication.

In the months of December and January, they went to the Sacramento Buddhist Church to help give typhoid vaccinations to all Japanese Americans in town. Six or seven thousand at least, Hara estimated.

"All lined up and here you're giving shots. And if they stayed too long in line, they'd get a second shot, because all you do is see arms," said Sugiyama. "We had people that were in line getting shots, and they'd go down a few steps and fall down and pass out because of shots. And if they got two shots...."

AUGUSTUS "GUS" TANAKA

On December 7, 1941, Gus Tanaka, the son of Hawaii-born Dr. Benjamin Tanaka, was at his family's Portland home. In his first year of premed studies at Reed College, Gus was eighteen years old.

"Dad was already out making hospital rounds," Gus remembered. "It was a Sunday morning, and he came home and had lunch. I guess it was about late afternoon; then the bell rang and two men were at the door. They said they wanted to talk to my father, and I told them he was out making rounds at the hospital, and I think he had one house call to make. They wanted to know when he'd be home. I said, 'Well, he'd come home.' He had called in and said he was going to be a little late for supper, and he'd be home for supper.... We didn't know who they were. Then we heard Dad come home to put his car away, but we never saw him. Well, it turned out that [they] were the FBI, and they were just hanging around waiting for him to show up. They took him away, and we never saw them....

"And then about twenty minutes later, these two same guys came. They identified themselves as FBI agents, and they explained that they had taken Dad away for security reasons, and they had to search the house. They came in and went through the house, everything. They just tore into the cupboards and things, closets and upstairs....

"It wasn't badly trashed, but they certainly didn't put it back the way they found it. Then they asked us if we had any weapons, any cameras, and they wanted to know if we had any radio transmitters. They asked us whether we had... radios... well, we only had one radio.

"Dad always had a revolver that he kept in the house for security. We told them, yes, we had one.... We had one little box of ammunition, and they wanted to know where the rest of it was. We said as far as we know, he kept them together and that's all he had. Then some old gentleman had paid off a medical bill with an old samurai sword. They wanted to know whether we had any swords, and they took all this away. They gave us a receipt for all these things....

"They didn't take the radio. They took everything else. They took all our cameras. Dad had an old Kodak movie camera; they took that. My mother had a sack of old Japanese magazines, written in Japanese. They took all those. Then my mother had some letters from her relatives in Japan, and they took all those.... But they gave us a receipt for it, and after the war, everything came back."

Gus surmised why his father had been taken. "There's no doubt that the FBI had a hit list of people who were prominent in the Japanese community. How they figured it out, I don't know. But Dad [was looked upon as] being one of the few college-educated people of his generation and being more or less of a community leader. You know the theory of cutting off the head so the body can't function? I think that was why. Because to my knowledge, Dad was not engaged in any subversive activity or anything like that. It came as a shock to me that they picked him up because what our training from him was: obey the law, be good citizens, study hard. He told us about the challenges that we would have to face as Japanese at that time. That you're going to have to work twice as hard to get half the recognition."

For a week to ten days, the Tanakas had no idea where their family patriarch was being held. "...then we were told that he was in the [Multnomah] County Jail. As I recall, they told us what day we could come visit him. So we all went down there at the time they said we could show up. That was an experience because...they took mug shots of us and fingerprinted us....then we visited him. It was like you see in the movies, the glass wall with a little porthole. They let us visit for about fifteen, twenty minutes, not very long. That's the last we saw of him."

Meanwhile, Gus's mother, Michiye (Yamada) Tanaka, was left to fend with the bills and taking care of the household on her own. "Then one day—I don't think we heard anything officially—I think it was through the grapevine, that they'd all been moved out. There were several weeks [before] we finally got a letter from him. They had moved them to another camp in Missoula, Montana. Basically, it was a camp for these nationals who happened to be caught in this country when the war broke out. Tourists and business people... were there, [they] were not really resident aliens, but visitors and people on business visas and so forth.

"We understood that the camp was terrible because these people couldn't get along with each other—the Germans, the Italians, and the Japanese groups. So they had to separate them, feed them separately, and house them separately and so forth."

His father's arrest took its toll on the Tanaka household. "[This] had a devastating effect on my ability to concentrate in school, and I just wasn't doing well. I remember going in to my faculty advisor and asking if maybe I should just withdraw and come back after the war or something.

"He said, 'No, no, we understand the situation. We'll take all this into consideration.'

"But around January, now this is only five or six weeks after Pearl Harbor, Dr. Arthur Scott, who was acting president of Reed College, who also happened to be the premed faculty advisor, called me into his office, and said, 'You know there's talk about evacuating all the Japanese from the coast. I really think we ought to start planning to get you transferred as soon as possible.'

"He asked me if I had any ideas of where to go. And I said, 'Well, I [have] no idea. Is there any place that would take me?'

"He said, 'Well, under the circumstances it might get a little touchy, but I'm sure there are places.'"

Through Scott's connections, Tanaka applied to the University of Minnesota, Oberlin College in Ohio, and finally Haverford College in Pennsylvania. Oberlin never responded, but the University of Minnesota president apologetically declined, citing the college's contract with the U.S. Air Force. "If the war ends, and you still have an interest in going to the University of Minnesota, write me personally, and we'll make sure that you'll get accepted as a transfer student," the president wrote.

Haverford College, on the other hand, warmly welcomed Tanaka—even communicating that a student wanted him as a roommate at the Quaker school. Reed College also did their part. "They waived the final exams for me. They waived all the terms papers. And they said, 'We are sending you out a bona fide having finished the freshman class.'"

Before Tanaka could leave for Pennsylvania, he learned that his family's plans had been changed. They were notified that they had to report to the Portland Assembly Center in May 1942.

JAMES N. YAMAZAKI

Unlike his upper classmates Dr. Henry Sugiyama and Dr. Shigeru Hara, James Yamazaki was still attending Marquette University in Milwaukee in 1941. He and his family back home in Los Angeles had sensed that war would break out in the tense Pacific, so Yamazaki had even volunteered for military service in the fall of 1941. He received his reserve commission a week before the bombing of Pearl Harbor.

Yamazaki's father, John Misao Yamazaki, was the pastor of the Japanese Episcopal Church, also known as St. Mary's, in Los Angeles' Uptown area. As clergy, he was considered a community leader and was visited by the authorities. "My mother told me that there would be a knock on the door, and the way they knocked, we knew even before going to it. She would say, 'FBI-*san* is at the door.'"

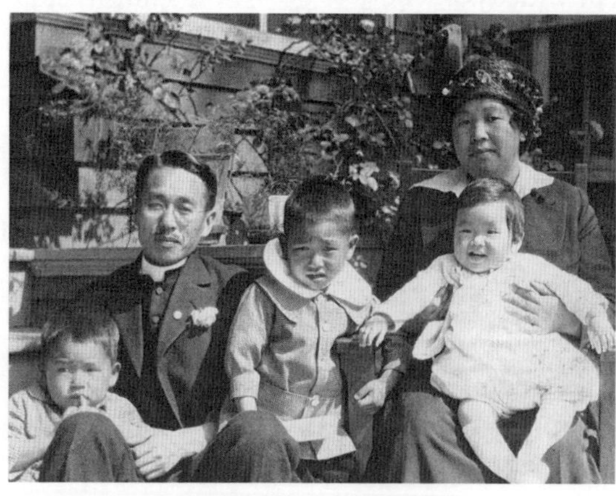

The Yamazaki family, Fall 1919, in front of the rectory next to St. Mary's Episcopal Mission. LEFT TO RIGHT: James Nobuo, 3 years; Rev. John Misao Yamazaki; John Michio, 5 years; Mary Tsune with Peter Tamio, about 9 months, in her arms.

But unlike the other Issei leaders, the minister was not taken into custody. Yamazaki believes that his father had told the FBI that he had a son in the U.S. Army. "The FBI did come to see me in Milwaukee," said Yamazaki. "... The same person that talked to my dad and [was] told that I was in the army. Of course, my dad didn't have my papers. [The FBI agent] came to Milwaukee and talked to me.... He was testing the veracity of my dad's statement."

MASAHARU RICHARD SETO

Born in San Francisco and raised in Sacramento, Dr. Richard Seto was in the middle of a residency at Yuba County Hospital when Japan bombed Pearl Harbor. A graduate of Marquette Medical School in 1941, Seto, also known as "Doc," had already completed his internship and residency at Sacramento County Hospital.

"It was during his residency at the Yuba County Hospital that he experienced discrimination, humiliation, and hurt," reported his wife Hideko "Deki" Seto. "Shortly after Pearl Harbor, an editorial in the local newspaper stated, 'We are having a Jap doctor delivering our babies,' with a caricature of a Japanese face, buck-toothed, and dark-rimmed glasses... a face, grinning stupidly. Then Doc went to the editor's office and was going to have him apologize. When he was ushered into the editor's office, he saw a disabled, crippled male sitting in a wheelchair. He thought, *Why approach him? This man has more problems than he can manage.*"

FRANK CHUMAN
MASAKO (KUSAYANAGI) MIURA
TOSHI YAMAMOTO

In 1941, twenty-five-year-old Toshi Yamamoto moved to Los Angeles from Seattle, Washington. There, she worked as the office manager for Dr. Yoshiye Togasaki, who had opened her own practice on Vermont Avenue in Uptown Los Angeles in July 1941 to provide consultation services. The doctor had spent six years at Los Angeles County General Hospital fulfilling a year internship and a five-year residency in communicable disease. For her residency, she was paid a generous $250 a month because of the "risk and responsibility."

Togasaki's eldest sister Kazue, who had completed her internship at Children's Hospital of San Francisco, had already started her own medical practice in 1935. Younger sister Teru, the seventh seventh-born child of Kikumatsu and Shige Togasaki, had earned her medical degree from the University of California. Three other sisters—Mitsuye, Chiye, and Yaye—had entered the nursing field.

Dr. James Goto was completing a surgical residency and Dr. Sakaye Shigekawa was fulfilling an obstetrical residency at Los Angeles County General Hospital, while Dr. Masako (Kusayanagi) Miura was accepted to the hospital's dermatology residency in July 1941. As part of her residency, Dr. Miura concentrated her studies on syphilology because "syphilis will mimic any disease. So if you know syphilis, you know medicine."

With the bombing of Pearl Harbor and the U.S. official entry into World War II, all Japanese Americans—including Shigekawa, Miura, Goto, and others—were called in by the hospital administrators.

"All the Japanese will have to go and will be discharged until ninety days after the war, and then they can be reinstated if they want to. But they'll be discharged until then," remembered Shigekawa.

Frank Chuman, a student at USC Law School, was also released from his part-time job at the Los Angeles County Probation Department. He, along with Dr. Tetsui "Tets" Watanabe, took note of the government's forcible removal of families from Terminal Island with only forty-eight-hour notice. Said Chuman, "A large number were coming up to Los Angeles and were being sheltered in the Nishi Hongwanji Temple [in Little Tokyo].... Tets Watanabe and I felt that they needed medical help. We were going to rent a storefront near Nishi Hongwanji. He would be the doctor to take care of them medically, and I was going to take care of the business part of this little private clinic that we were going to organize."

The clinic, however, failed to materialize because of President Franklin D. Roosevelt's Executive Order 9066. The presidential order authorized the removal and imprisonment of individuals by the War Department. Soon after, proclamations announced that the West

Coast would be divided into military zones and that those of Japanese ancestry, both alien and "non-alien," would be forced to move from their homes. For 110,000 of these people, detention camps spread throughout the nation's interior would be their eventual destination.

Dr. John Bowden of the United States Public Health Service, seeking to recruit volunteers for Manzanar, located in California's Owens Valley, held a meeting for health professionals in Little Tokyo. Apparently at this meeting, Watanabe had recommended Chuman for the job of hospital administrator.

There were still many answered questions. "We didn't know the status of what was going to happen," remembered Toshi Yamamoto. "Being that Dr. Togasaki was with contagious diseases, she knew that small pox and typhoid shots would have to be given. And she went out of her way to contact the army... to find out what the program would be. Whether they knew it [or not], they didn't tell her.... But she never got a satisfactory answer."

After their release from the county hospital, Goto and Miura, who had just married, decided to open their own practice in an office in Miura's father's building in downtown Los Angeles. The news of their medical practice spread through word of mouth, and soon patients were coming in. About six weeks later, a government visitor from Washington, D.C., Dr. G.D. Carlyle Thompson, came to talk to them. "He wanted us to go into the camps and help out with the patients over there," explained Miura. "I said, 'What kind of salary are we going to get? Will we get public health wages?'

"He said, "Yes, I think so.'

"I said, 'Well, will I get the same first or second grade that the public health officers get?"

"He said, 'Yes, you'll get that.'"

Togasaki was also finally notified, given only forty-eight hours to settle her personal matters. She was promised by authorities that if she went to Manzanar, the rest of the Togasaki family would be sent to the same California camp. (That promise was never fulfilled. Teru and Susumu were incarcerated at Poston, Arizona, while Chiye and Kazue were sent to Tule Lake, California. Kikumatsu, Sugi, and Shinobu spent a portion of the war years in Topaz, Utah.) Yoshiye

Togasaki met others at a church and drove up to Manzanar in sedans as part of a caravan. As Togasaki and her friend were driving their own cars, "I had vacuum cleaners, typewriters, and things of this sort, even cooking utensils."

Togasaki, in fact, had spent time in the Owens Valley. "That was my vacation ground. I used to go there all the time for my vacations. One of my interns lived at Independence. I knew the area and it was beautiful. The weather was not as forbidding as the desert of Arizona and Utah."

But once the caravan arrived, Togasaki discovered that her experience would be very different from her previous sojourns as a tourist. Toshi Yamamoto recalled, "When [Togasaki] went up there, the hospital part was not even ready.... Just a bunch of straw and mattresses you were supposed to fill up. She was very annoyed with that. She said, 'When you're going to bring thousands of civilians, you do your work and get some of it done because you're uprooting people that have never left their own house.'"

Miura also discovered that government promises of wages would not be met. As she observed, "when we got in, you're nothing but an evacuee."

KATSUMI JAMES NAKADATE

Dr. Katsumi James Nakadate was a second-year head resident at Eloise, Michigan, a town outside of Detroit, in 1941. He had earlier joined the U.S. Army Reserve and had received orders to report to the military after his first year of residency. But his hospital had requested that Nakadate be allowed to complete his second year because of his senior resident status. Everything changed on December 7, 1941.

"Pearl Harbor happened on a Sunday," said Nakadate. "On Monday morning, the hospital called and said, "There's a couple of people here to see you, and they're in the medical director's office.

"I went there, who do you think they were, the two men?...FBI, and they knew about me because, you can't believe this, the person in the FBI office in Detroit...was a fellow Eagle Scout from Portland, Oregon. He became an FBI man, and he had told them about me, all about me. So when I went into the office, they said, 'We know all about you, doctor.'

"So for the rest of that time, I used to go eat with them, with the FBI fellows in Detroit. Isn't that something?"

ROBERT S. KINOSHITA

On March 27, 1941, Dr. Robert S. Kinoshita, a captain with the U.S. Army and district surgeon of the Medford District CCC, was named as an examining physician to one of the districts within the Douglas County Selective Service board in Oregon. "He was serving in that position when Pearl Harbor was attacked," said his son Richard. "Upon the declaration of war against Japan by the United States, my father asked for active duty. At that time, there was curfew for Japanese-ancestry people. On that particular night, he was to teach a nursing class that was another one of his duties that he did. He was supposed to teach a Red Cross class to registered nurses at one of the hospitals. Because of the curfew, he called the nearest FBI office, identified himself, and was told that they knew all about him, that he was to go ahead and carry out his medical duties as before, despite the curfew, which he did."

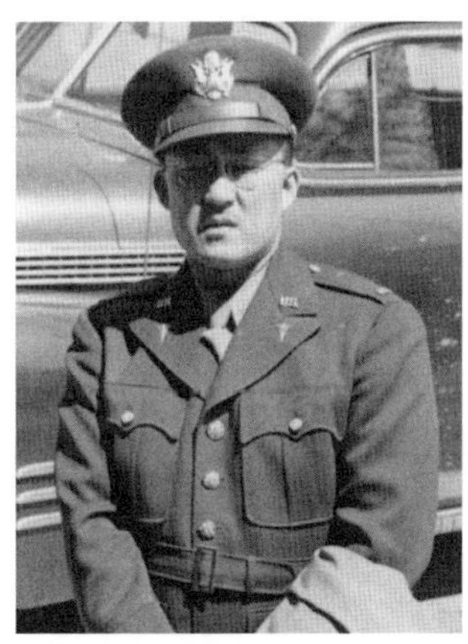

Dr. Katsumi J. Nakadate in uniform, East Chicago, May 6, 1943.

After the presidential exclusion order and announcements that those of Japanese ancestry had to leave portions of the West Coast, Kinoshita received an order to report to Fort Omaha, Nebraska. "That would have gotten our family off the West Coast. They immediately sold their largest possessions, packed up what was left, and took them to Portland, Oregon, for storage. By that time, Executive Order 9066 was in full order. While they were storing their possessions, apparently someone in the JACL [Japanese American Citizens League] saw he was in the area [and] asked the WRA to assign him as a doctor at the Portland Assembly Center.

"The WRA contacted the army and had my father's orders cancelled. That meant that he had to go into camp, along with my brother. When they did report to the assembly center, the WRA would not allow my mother to enter because she's Caucasian. She was told that, strangely enough, she was pregnant at the time with me, that when her baby was born, I would have to go into the camp, but she would not be allowed. There was no way she was going to comply with that.

"She was given a piece of paper to sign, saying that she would abide by the same rules as the Japanese Americans, that she would never sue the United States government over the matter. Then she was allowed to enter. My father, my brother, and my pregnant mother were put in a horse stall."

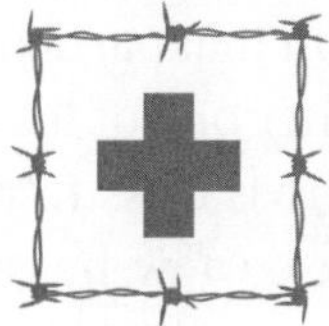

4. TEMPORARY DETENTION CENTERS

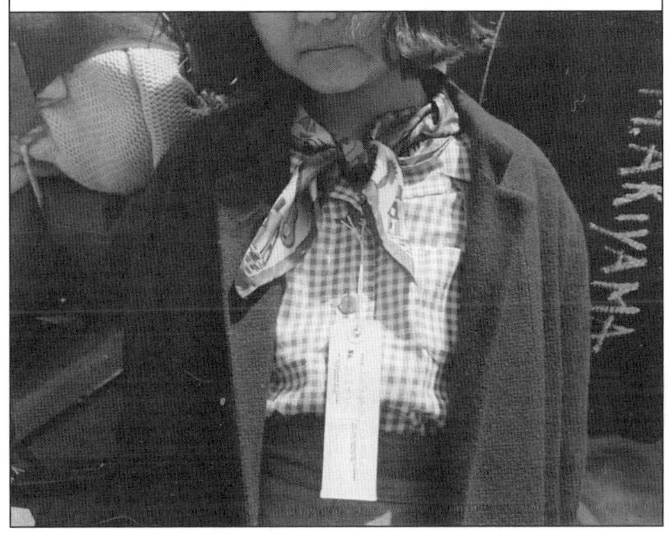

I remember going out on a number of barracks calls in an ambulance with a Dr. Kuroiwa, and carrying his doctor bag with me. That was my first introduction to a home call.

—Robert Obi, MD, who was an extern at Santa Anita Assembly Center

By the end of March 1942, the government established sixteen temporary detention centers in fairgrounds, racetracks, and parks. These centers were located in California (Fresno, Owens Valley, Marysville, Merced, Pinedale, Pomona, Sacramento, Salinas, Santa Anita, Stockton, Tanforan, Tulare, Turlock), Washington (Puyallup), Oregon (Portland), and Arizona (Mayer). More than 110,000 Japanese Americans were forcibly removed from their homes and moved into horse stables and other buildings unfit for human habitation, putting them at risk of typhoid and other contagious infections. Doctors and other medical personnel fulfilled an important role in administering inoculations to prevent the spread of disease in cramped quarters. These temporary detention centers were in operation until November 1942, when the inmates were transferred to permanent detention.

HENRY IWAO SUGIYAMA
MASAMICHI "MAC" SUZUKI

Although Dr. Mac Suzuki and his medical school classmate and friend Dr. Ed Nishimura were not licensed, they were still ordered to be part of the hospital staff of the Sacramento Assembly Center, also known as Walerga, in Northern Sacramento. Dr. George Iki, an Issei surgeon educated in San Francisco at the UC Medical School, was in charge of organizing the medical team. Iki had been one of the Suzuki family doctors. "I had developed quite a few boils in my youth," said Suzuki, "and [Dr. Iki] lanced them. Finally, he had a bacteriologist culture my infection, which was a staphylococcus [species], and had a vaccine made for me. It worked because after the treatment I didn't develop any boils."

Also on hand was one of Suzuki's other doctors, Masaatsu Harada, another graduate of UC Medical School. He was an Issei born in 1899.

"Walerga had no hospital but a small clinic," said Suzuki. "We had no major sick patients. All I can recall about this period was that we had a food poisoning [outbreak] one night, and we ran around giving paregoric.... Spoonfuls. People were running back and forth to the outdoor latrine. It was one of those army-type of the open johnny."

Dr. Henry Sugiyama also recalled these "open johnnies": "They had outhouses with three holes on a plank in a little room, no flush." There were no separate toilet facilities for men and women. "And when they had diarrhea, [the women] were waiting in line for [the men] to leave so they could get into the place."

Sugiyama, who had entered Walerga Assembly Center with only his small medical bag, five dollars, and a suitcase with four changes of clothes, also was struck by the primitiveness of the Walerga hospital, which had no beds. Sugiyama had a personal stake in the condition of the hospital, because his sister was having complications with her pregnancy. "She had toxemia, elevated blood pressure and swelling," he recalled.

"I said, 'I want to send her to the [county] hospital because she's toxic. If you don't do something, we're going to have trouble.'"

"... [The white administrator] said, 'You're going to Tule Lake in a few weeks, so why don't we—you—bear with her.'"

"I said, 'I can't wait that long.'"

"[The administrator] said, 'Well, you'll just have to.'"

"So her baby died."

SHIGERU HARA

Dr. Shigeru Hara and his wife were sent to the smaller of the two temporary detention centers in the Sacramento area, Marysville, commonly known as Arboga. At its peak, Arboga had close to 2,500 inmates, in contrast to 4,700 in Walerga.

"The army had requested barracks for everybody, but they built the barracks [with] wooden cots, the two-tier cots. The army came and checked that and said they had to take them all out. So they took all those cots out of every barracks and piled them up, and they were burning them. They gave us army cots instead.... So everybody used to go out to the dump and pick up that lumber and make things out of it. The only thing is, the nails were burned, and they were very soft. My brother and I used to have to straighten them out and nail very carefully. Otherwise they'd bend. So we picked up that lumber. My older brother, who's pretty handy, built a delivery table for us, because there was none in the hospital."

HOMER YASUI

Homer Yasui had been a senior at Hood River High School in north central Oregon when he and his remaining family members received the notice that they had to move. His father Masuo had been already taken by the FBI and was held first at the Multnomah County Jail before being moved to Fort Missoula, Montana. Yasui, his mother, and younger sister were all sent to Pinedale Assembly Center, a few miles north of Fresno in California's San Joaquin Valley.

"We were surrounded on two sides with fig orchards, and I'd never seen fig trees before," described Yasui. "...But the main thing that was most impressive about it [was that] it was hot, and it was crowded. Even more impressive for me was seeing so many Japanese in one place. I'd never seen that many before. There were over four thousand of us in this one camp, in an area of about one square mile.

"It originally was a sawmill when they'd haul the logs down from the Sierra Nevadas. Then later on the sawmill was abandoned, and apparently they used to have sawmill workers living where we were housed. They tore that down because they had some of the plumbing in there already. They built barracks there and put us where the previous lumberyard employees had lived."

Seventeen-year-old Yasui applied for a job as an orderly at the Pinedale medical clinic, which he described as a "rinky-dink infirmary, a temporary setup." The infirmary consisted of a single standard barracks, 120 by 20 feet. "It was kind of a temporary care station, almost like a medical aid station more than anything else because any of the seriously ill patients were transported to Fresno General Hospital." Because the number of young people wanting positions as orderlies and nurse's aides exceeded the number of openings, Yasui was given another task. "What they did with me is they gave me a bucket of lime and made me a sanitary inspector."

"In Pinedale, we had no flush toilets," said Yasui. "There were showers, and there [were] laundry facilities, but no flush toilets. They were all privies. I don't know why. Anyway, it wouldn't have made much difference I think because I don't think they had the septic tanks to handle it. I remember some of the soapy, scummy water, gray water from the laundry would run out in the streets there. You know how that smell is, a sour smell."

For $8 a month, Yasui inspected these "one- and two-holers": "I'd just rap on the door, and I was supposed to dump lime into these toilets." Later he also helped deliver bottled milk prepared by student nurses to new mothers. "In those days, most of the young mothers were Issei, and a lot of the Issei women could not speak English or understand English very well. Some of them not at all.

"So [out] of necessity, whoever was delivering the milk would have a list of which stations and which women [could] get the milk for their baby because it wasn't that easy to get. So usually we'd go off, and we'd call out the name of 'Mrs. Yamada,' and she'd say, 'Here.' So we'd hand out her one or two bottles....

"One day we were delivering the milk, and it happened it was my turn to call out the name. So I handed out the milk, and I asked this woman [who] came in front of me to pick up the milk for her baby: '*Nanjoo nan desu ka*?' (That's colloquial for, 'What is your name, please?')

"Well, I found out later... that wasn't good Japanese at all. In fact, it was very crude. Because the real way to ask what a person's name would be: '*Onamae wa nan desu ka*?'

"But I didn't know that because I was speaking the Japanese that I'd learned at home. The interesting thing about that is my mother was a junior-high graduate, and she was a teacher, and so she knew standard Japanese. But what I didn't realize or know, was that at home my mother and father spoke Okayama-*ben*, which is a dialect, a prefectural dialect. It's not standard Japanese, but that's what I was speaking.

"So when we started our ride in the jeep back to the infirmary, the driver and the driver's aide asked me, 'What did you say to that woman?'

"I said, '*Nanjoo nani desu ka*?'

"And they laughed. They said, 'That's not the way you ask a person what their name is. You're supposed to say, '*Onamae wa nan desu ka*?'

"But I never knew that, and to this day, I'm kind of mad at my folks for not telling us that they weren't speaking standard Japanese. But that was a funny experience."

He also enjoyed the fellowship of the doctors, especially those who had transferred to Pinedale from nearby Tulare Assembly Center near Fresno. "One of them was Hugo O'Konogi, whose father [Bunkuro O'Konogi] also was a doctor, but [the father] stayed in the Fresno camp. Then the other doctor's name was... Dr. Kanai, and he was the uncle of a student nurse who all of us were deeply in love with," said Yasui.

O'Konogi, who had a prewar medical practice in Fresno, was notable since he spelled his last name "like an Irishman would: capital O, apostrophe, capital K." "He was a very impressive, very interesting fellow. He had a beautiful baritone voice, and sometimes he'd sing for us," remembered Yasui.

WILLIAM SATO

Back in Tulare Assembly Center was William Sato, another young Nisei who also observed the "wonders" of sanitation at the temporary detention center. "The toilet facility was just like a huge glorified hole in the ground... except that they had a four-by-eight-by-knee high bench, and they had four or five holes on one side, four or five holes in the back and only about that much space [indicating a foot] between each. In the first couple of weeks, we all had diarrhea so it was standing room only.... They had a funny flushing system. There was sheet metal on the bottom, and it tilted to one side. On one side, they had a big tank that kept filling all the time with water. Then after a certain time, it would tilt and then go into a funnel device and come dashing down and splash. At the end, it would splash up like that, so everyone was doing this. They'd wait for the flushing noise, and then they'd stand up. It was like a ballet."

EMI (SOMEKAWA) BECKWITH

Portland-born Emi (Somekawa) Beckwith had become a nurse in Oregon, graduating from nurse's training at Emanuel Hospital in 1939. Three years later, she was married and a mother of an infant and pregnant with another child. Their family was sent to live in a horse stall in Portland Assembly Center, yet Beckwith still agreed to work at the hospital because "when you have a profession like that, you feel like you're needed."

On her first day of work at the hospital, Beckwith noticed that there were at least ten patients, including her father-in-law, who had suffered a stroke before the incarceration. There were few supplies or instruments, aside from an emergency kit to treat lacerations and other minor injuries. "I didn't think we had enough emergency type of instruments, like if someone came in with a fracture. Of course, we had no X-ray.... No X-ray at all. Those people, if we thought they had a fracture, even a finger, we couldn't tell.... they just put a splint on, and they just let it go at that. Of course, if it's a real bad fracture, leg fracture, or something like that, I think they sent them out... in an ambulance to Multnomah County Hospital." Multnomah County

Hospital was approximately fifteen miles away. Although there were much closer private hospitals, the government hadn't bothered to contract services from them and used only public medical facilities.

Sheets were limited, and the bath and laundry facilities were inadequate. With only three doctors and five to six nurses, a larger problem was the lack of trained personnel, especially nurse's aides. "In one incident, a patient had a seizure while his temperature was being taken. As a result, he had bit into the thermometer."

"Well, we need to completely wash him out; get all that mercury out," Beckwith and the other medical staff decided. But the patient was already unconscious and he died soon afterward from his seizures.

An epidemic also resulted from possible food poisoning. "We had a case of diarrhea that was just pathetic. Not enough bathroom facilities, and I was one (affected). It was awful. About every ten minutes I had to run to the bathroom, and then you get to the bathroom, and there's no place to go because the places are full. It was just an awful thing. We figured it was Vienna sausage. They served that day after day after day, and everybody got sick."

Pregnant with her second child, Beckwith attempted to eat as nutritionally as possible. As there was no baby food for her infant daughter, she attempted to make a gruel out of leftover rice from the mess hall on a portable electric plate that she had brought with her to the temporary detention center. When she was finally ready to deliver in August, she was sent to her former training site, Emanuel Hospital instead of Multnomah County Hospital. "With my first delivery, I had almost thirty-six hours of labor. Dr. Schauffer, who was my obstetrician, sent a note to the executive director of the assembly center that whenever I start labor that I am to be sent to Emanuel Hospital. There was a note from the doctor. They went along with that, so I had no problem."

While the delivery was smooth, a complication arose upon their return to the temporary detention center. Her newborn son couldn't take formula or powdered milk. "He was losing weight," Beckwith said. "Finally, I don't know who, somebody said, 'Well, why don't you try this Special Morning milk?'

"So I said, 'Okay, if I can get some.'"

Fortunately, with Beckwith's connections with nurses outside of camp, she was able to purchase the special milk. "So I got some, and he made it okay."

FRED FUJIKAWA
ROBERT OBI
SAKAYE SHIGEKAWA

Robert Obi was a second-year student at USC Medical School during the outbreak of the war with the Pacific. He was the nephew of Dr. George Takeyama, the pioneering physician whose name was used to secure the Boyle Heights property for the Japanese Hospital in Los Angeles. Obi's father had been a businessman and proprietor of a store in Little Tokyo, yet Obi still had to work at Three Star Produce in Los Angeles to raise money for his tuition at USC. Due to the forced removal of Japanese Americans, he had to cut his education short. He and his family were first sent to Santa Anita Assembly Center, a former horse racetrack in Arcadia.

"When we first got there, we were fortunate because...we obtained one of the newer barracks that had been built on the auto parking area. Many people were sent over [to] the stable area....they had to live in the horse stables. And the majority of cases, although [the stables] were said to be whitewashed and painted, the paint practically was rubbed off by the manure that was already plastered onto the walls. The smell was still there, and the manure was still there and flaking off...that was one of the sore points of the stable area. They eventually were able to get someone to come in and scrape off as much as they could and painted over. I doubt if that was a routine thing they did."

Dr. Sakaye Shigekawa was one of those assigned to the horse stables. After being dismissed from her obstetrical residency at Los Angeles County General Hospital, Shigekawa joined the staff of Seaside Memorial Hospital in Long Beach, only to receive immediate notice that she, along with the Terminal Islanders, needed to leave the area and go into Santa Anita Assembly Center. "I just didn't believe our government would do that," she said. "So when I was

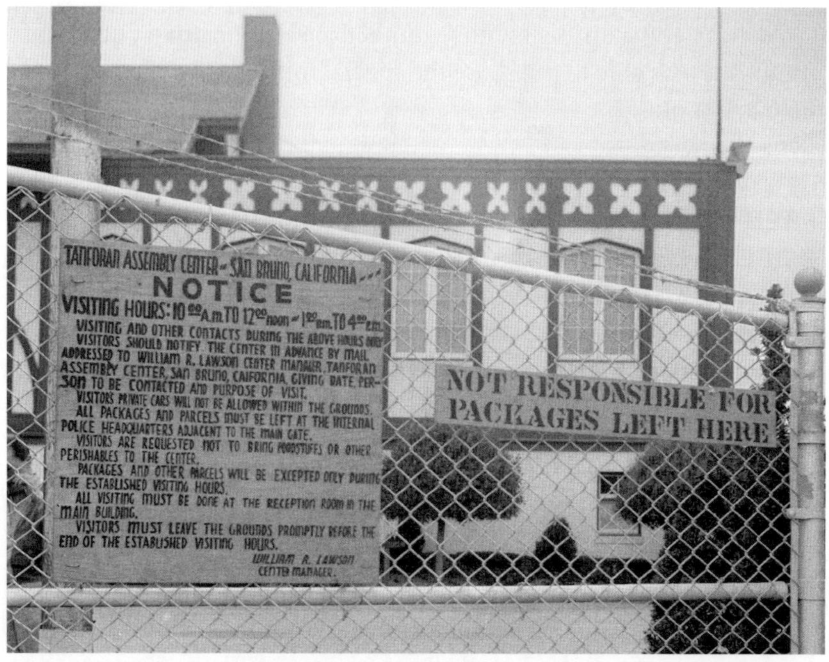

TANFORAN ASSEMBLY CENTER – SAN BRUNO, CALIFORNIA
NOTICE
VISITING HOURS: 10 A.M. TO 12 NOON – 1 P.M. TO 4 P.M.
VISITING AND OTHER CONTACTS DURING THE ABOVE HOURS ONLY
VISITORS SHOULD NOTIFY THE CENTER IN ADVANCE BY MAIL ADDRESSED TO WILLIAM R. LAWSON CENTER MANAGER, TANFORAN ASSEMBLY CENTER, SAN BRUNO, CALIFORNIA, GIVING DATE, PERSON TO BE CONTACTED AND PURPOSE OF VISIT.
VISITORS PRIVATE CARS WILL NOT BE ALLOWED WITHIN THE GROUNDS.
ALL PACKAGES AND PARCELS MUST BE LEFT AT THE INTERNAL POLICE HEADQUARTERS ADJACENT TO THE MAIN GATE.
VISITORS ARE REQUESTED NOT TO BRING FOODSTUFFS OR OTHER PERISHABLES TO THE CENTER.
PACKAGES AND OTHER PARCELS WILL BE EXCEPTED ONLY DURING THE ESTABLISHED VISITING HOURS.
ALL VISITING MUST BE DONE AT THE RECEPTION ROOM IN THE MAIN BUILDING.
VISITORS MUST LEAVE THE GROUNDS PROMPTLY BEFORE THE END OF THE ESTABLISHED VISITING HOURS.
WILLIAM R. LAWSON
CENTER MANAGER.
NOT RESPONSIBLE FOR
PACKAGES LEFT HERE
A sign at the main entrance of the Tanforan Assembly Center, San Bruno, California.

in camp I felt very bitter about it.... I was half the time crying and half the time resenting everything that was done to me. Later on the doctors formed a clinic in the compound there, under the bleachers. [The Nisei doctors] started a clinic."

Dr. Norman Kobayashi, a Los Angeles Nisei doctor, served as chief medical officer. Shigekawa reported to the clinic. "I was so unhappy, and I didn't know any of those doctors, so I'd sit there. I guess I was depressed, and I thought, 'Well, gee, if this is the life I have to lead I'd rather be dead.' I was very unhappy, and so Dr. Kobayashi stopped and talked to me.

"He said, "You know, just learn to accept this and just go along with it, because there's nothing you can do.' ...

"So I went along, then I started to see some patients, and then at least I could forget where I was. But I was very bitter. I'd see kids marching, waving the flag and all that, and I thought, 'What does that flag mean? It's just a rag.' I used to feel so reverent when I saw the flag waving... [and now] I thought, 'Well, it's just a symbol.'"

Besides Kobayashi, Dr. Fred Fujikawa also extended his friendship to Shigekawa. But it was not always easy to serve patients under the camp conditions. "Some of them didn't seem to appreciate what was done for them.

"And I told Dr. Kobayashi, 'Gee, I don't think I like this.'

"And he said, "Well, remember these people are going through this trauma just like you." And he told me, 'Just be sympathetic with them, and just listen and take care of them.'"

While Nikkei doctors in Central and Northern California organized to immunize everyone in their areas before they entered camp, most of the Southern Californians received their inoculations upon arrival to temporary detention. "And they'd get sick because of high fever and diarrhea and so forth," said Fujikawa. "I've seen them line up to go to the toilet, you know. And they would faint. A lot. It was about the saddest thing I'd ever seen in camp."

Shigekawa continued to persevere under these conditions, but in the beginning, did not carry on much conversation with the patients. She was still relatively inexperienced and couldn't speak Japanese that well. She was assigned to the dermatology department and treated individuals with skin rashes. "In those days, we really didn't have medication to take care of it. So they had one thing called gentian violet, so you painted them. Everything they had, I painted with gentian violet. So it went around that if they had that purple on them, they had seen me."

Among the young externs assisting Shigekawa was Obi. "Being in my sophomore year, I was already introduced into taking histories, physical examinations," he said. "Dr. Shigekawa was very instrumental in teaching me a lot of dermatology in those days because the camp population was very prone to allergic types of dermatitis coming from the camouflage netting project that was going on.... That was a huge netting that was suspended from the grandstand, into which was woven the different colored gunny-sack type material to make a camouflage pattern on this netting, which was then shipped out to the military areas to cover...tanks, guns, airplanes, and whatever they wanted to camouflage and prevent detection.... That was on one of the projects to keep the evacuees busy."

Dust would arise from this gunny-sack material, thereby irritating the workers' skin. As a result, gentian violet, also used for trench mouth, was used to alleviate the dermatitis, Obi explained.

Obi received his first initiation into conducting house calls in camp. "I remember going out on a number of barracks calls in an ambulance with a Dr. Kuroiwa and carrying his doctor bag with me. That was my first introduction to a home call."

Shigekawa, meanwhile, wanted more of a challenge than painting patients with gentian violet. "You know," she said to Kobayashi and Fujikawa, "you folks are doing surgery...and I'm just doing this. I think it's only right that you let me do other things."

The senior doctors concurred, and before long, Shigekawa was assisting in the operating room and delivering babies. The medical equipment and ambulances seemed to date back twenty years to World War I.

"Before World War II, we didn't have any really good medicines to take care of anything. Just two handfuls of medicine, and we could memorize all of them." On hand were aspirin; ammonium chloride, a diuretic for the heart; and theophylline, used to treat asthma. For infection, the camp doctors had sulfa drugs.

Shigekawa was impressed with the diagnostic skills of the more experienced doctors. "I always admired them because they were very conscientious about it, and our diagnosis was correct most of the time," she said.

There were, however, tragic incidents, usually resulting from shoddy equipment or limited resources. In one incident, a mother began bleeding after giving birth. "We...did everything possible but she hemorrhaged, and no matter what we did she kept on hemorrhaging. She had five children, and this was her sixth, and she died." Since the Santa Anita clinic had no blood, no transfusions could be administered. "At least if we started a transfusion, it might have been helpful. It might have kept her alive long enough till we found where the source was."

Shigekawa also remembered an epidemic of diarrhea that broke out in Santa Anita. "These patients were running to the latrine, and people were lined up; they couldn't hardly make it. The latrines were open, and most of these people were not used to going to the toilet in public. So it was quite an experience at that time."

It was only a matter of time before fears fueled rumors. "They were sure that we were being poisoned.... 'This is it. The government's going to poison us.'

"Some of them had that feeling, so we had to tell them no, it wasn't, that public health was going to come out and see why this happened, because it was the food naturally. It was food that was standing too long."

FRANK CHUMAN
YOSHIYE TOGASAKI
TOSHI YAMAMOTO

When Frank Chuman, Dr. James Goto, and Fumiko Gohata arrived in Manzanar on March 21, 1942, they were assigned to two units within a barracks at Block Seven. "That was a makeshift, make-do facility, basically for minor surgery and compulsory, mandatory immunization of everybody that came in, that was a must. We didn't want any epidemics spreading around," said Chuman.

At this time, Manzanar was a temporary detention center operated by the army-controlled Wartime Civil Control Administration (WCCA). In the early days, the camp had little medical amenities. In the very beginning, in fact, Chuman and Goto slept on one side of the hospital barracks, their iron cot and straw mattresses hidden from view behind a blanket hanging from a wire strung across the room.

Inside the makeshift hospital there were an operating table, wash basin, hotplate, and a few instruments. It was Frank Chuman's responsibility to organize an infrastructure for the one-barrack hospital and order supplies. "Very quickly," he said, "I set up not a complicated table of organization for the entire hospital—a means to get things done. I had no training [or] experience with hospital administration, with nit-picky procedures, go-by-the-book. [I was] completely pragmatic."

Dr. Yoshiye Togasaki also didn't waste any time. With the help of a public health nurse, Togasaki began her mission to vaccinate more than ten thousand people for various communicable diseases, such as small pox, typhoid, para-typhoid, tetanus, and diphtheria. "DPT was something we had to get ourselves," said Togasaki regarding the three-in-one vaccine that is usually given to children to protect against diphtheria, tetanus, and pertussis, a bacterial infection that causes whopping cough. "The government wasn't providing it. They had tetanus and diphtheria but not the whooping cough. The Navy then was accustomed to handling young, healthy boys ... I said, 'But [these are] children. [It] is necessary.'"

Togasaki got in touch with a female researcher at Stanford University to obtain pertussis immunizations. "We got it eventually despite what the Navy thought. The fact [is] that it avoided epidemics." During the first month of the center's operation, 14,750 typhoid inoculations and 6,968 small pox were administered.

"I took my equipment with me," explained Togasaki. "First of all, we had very few nurses and except for the one public health nurse who was with me, the rest of them were in demand at the hospital. They preferred to work there because nurses aren't accustomed to working in field work. They are clinic and hospital hospital-trained. We had to train the young girls in cleaning and sharpening the needles after every use. Later on we had access to autoclaving at the hospital. We had no infections as a result of it, fortunately."

Working with Dr. Togasaki in Manzanar, Toshi Yamamoto was in charge of monitoring and checking immunization records. "[I got] the names [on] the cards of people who were to appear that day for their shots. Because if they had missed their day of the third or the second inoculation, the ambulance driver had a list of names, and would go out and tell them that you have to report for your second shot today."

Some internees, especially certain Kibei (those born in America but educated in Japan), did not respond well to Togasaki's reminders. Togasaki, who was always dressed in jodhpur riding pants while she went on her rounds, could not speak Japanese well. "She told them that if they didn't show up, she was going to get the ambulance to bring them up there."

"Oh no, you're not," the internees retorted.

Final Issue September 12, 1942 TOTALIZER

TANFORAN MEDICAL CENTER

Already 34 doctors, nurses, and other medical specialists have left Tanforan for relocation. More will be going with each new contingent of evacuees. And, with the general clinic handling only emergency cases from today, the last days of the Medical Center rapidly approach.

But the residents, who watched it grow from an embryo of 3 empty barracks to an efficient hospital unit, won't soon forget its accomplishments, under conditions far from ideal. Nor will they forget soon the men and women who made it the finest medical lay-out in the assembly centers, in the judgement of WCCA officials and U.S. Public Health authorities.

Resident chief of staff was Dr. K. Kitagawa, who succeeded Dr. Hajime Uyeyama when the latter departed for Tule Lake. A member of the American Medical Association, he has practiced medicine for 23 years, after graduating from the Stanford Medical School.

Working with him were 9 doctors, each with a forte: Kazue Togasaki, obstetrics; Eugenia Fujita, pediatrics; Masayuki Hara, cardiac cases; Kunisada Kiyasu, pediatrics; Benjamin Kondo, communicable disease and cardiac cases; Koichi Shimizu, hospital; John Teshima, clinic; California Ushiro, chest; and Paul Yamauchi, cardiac cases and clinic.

Head nurse was Masaye Mori, who, after graduating from U C Nursing School, was appointed supervisor of surgery at U C Hospital, a position she held for 3½ years. Assisting her were 8 registered nurses, 7 student nurses, 30 nurses' aides and 6 orderlies, constituting 26% of the hospital personnel.

Total number of persons employed by the Medical Center, including those working in the pharmacy, laboratory and diet and formulae kitchens, was 188.

Perhaps the man most responsible for the administrative success was Don Wild, superintendent of the Center infirmary, who was formerly supervisor of medical welfare at San Mateo Community Hospital. Since his appointment, about 2½ months ago, Wild initiated improvements in the dental and optometry clinics, enlarged the laboratory, and instituted an office routine patterned after regular hospital procedure.

Close coordination between the various units resulted in an average of 200 treatments per day, about 1000 to 1300 a week. Between April 30 and Sept. 4, more than 35,000 cases were diagnosed or treated by the general clinic. Most common ailments were diarrhea, sprains and colds.

But the general clinic wasn't the only busy department around the Medical Center. The dental clinic averaged 80 to 90 patients daily, and was so busy that appointments were made a month ahead. Up to the beginning of this week, it had treated 4777 cases, including 610 extractions, 854 temporary fillings and 555 permanent fillings.

The optometry clinic, before closing, issued approximately 1000 prescriptions. Of the average of [illegible]0 persons who daily visited the clinic, 3 or 4 walked in with broken glasses. The usual jobs were

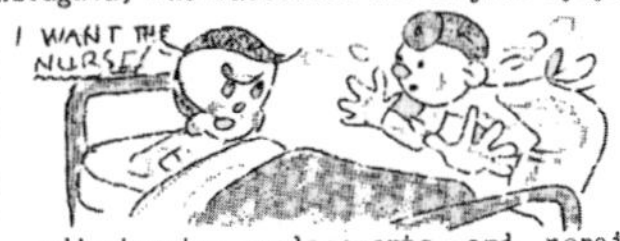

adjustments, replacements and repairs.

Another vital cog in the Tanforan medical machinery was the maternity ward, where 47 of the 52 babies born to Center residents were delivered. The ward contains pre-natal and post-natal rooms and constitutes one complete maternity set-up. The usual term of stay for a mother and her baby was 14 days, but many mothers were reluctant about leaving. "I don't blame some of the issei mothers," said Obstetrician Kazue Togasaki, "with nurses and fellow patients they can speak Japanese to, it's better than the hospitals outside."

Beside her job as obstetrician, Dr. Togasaki headed the Center-wide immunization program. With 22 girls assisting (a number which was later cut to 12), she vaccinated 99.8% of the Center population, sometimes going to the homes of those who didn't show up at the hospital. Immunization against typhoid, small pox and diptheria was mandatory; pertussis and tuberculin tests, voluntary. At present the immunization department is completing its records for forwarding to relocation.

With the medical program ramifying into so many clinics and departments, it was necessary to establish a central agency for testing and analyzing. This was provided by the laboratory, which obtained a blood count and urine test from every patient to register in the hospital. Other tests conducted by Technicians Yoshiko Kanzaki, Hisa Sugimoto and Yoshio Sato included appendicitis exams, Wassermans, sedimentation, blood typing and sputum tests.

But even with these facilities, many cases were beyond the scope of the Medical Center. About 396 cases were transferred to San Mateo Community Hospital.

In relocation, there won't be a big hospital like that to which "hard" cases may be conveniently sent. But observers who have watched the Medical Center staff at work feel that it has the ability and the guts to meet the challenge of administering to the needs of a pioneer community.

News article about Kazue Togasaki in the *Tanforan Totalizer*.

INSTRUCTIONS ON EVACUATION TO TULE LAKE

The people listed below are hereby directed to be prepared to leave this Center for Relocation Center at Tule Lake on Friday June 26 1942, and must report to the NORTH END of the INDUCTION BUILDING at ~~[illegible]~~ P.M. prepared to check out and board buses for train. 5:50 pm

NAME	U.S.E.S. No.	I.D. No.	ADDRESS
Kambara, George May Kusui	6508	506	3-6-C

PRELIMINARY PREPARATIONS

On Thursday June 25 commencing at 8:00 A.M., the interior guards will conduct an inspection of all property in your apartments. Immediately thereafter, you will pack all personal property EXCEPT BED ROLLS, TRUNKS, and HAND BAGGAGES for loading into freight cars. This freight must be placed OUTSIDE of your apartments ready for tagging and pick-up by truck within two hours after inspection. All property such as sewing machines, large radios, and anything that may be damaged in transit must be crated.

On Friday June 26 between 8:00 and 9:00 A.M., ALL FEDERAL BLANKETS must be returned to warehouse No. 1 in order to clear charges against your account. By 10:00 A.M. all Bed Rolls, Trunks and Hand Baggages must be packed and placed OUTSIDE your apartment ready for tagging and pick-up by truck. It will be permissible to carry small bundles and overnight hand baggage into the train.

On the day of movement, an early dinner will be served to those leaving at kitchen # 6 at 4:30 P.M.

N. L. Bican
N. L. Bican, Manager
Marysville Assembly Center
W.C.C.A.

Instructions for move from Marysville to Tule Lake for the Kambara family.

Yamamoto remembered one man as saying, "Just because you've got riding pants on, don't think you're all that."

MASAKO (KUSAYANAGI) MIURA

As the hospital was housed in a regular barracks, there were definite limitations, observed Dr. Masako (Kusayanagi) Miura, who joined the first convoy of volunteers from Los Angeles to Manzanar. "We found out that there was sometimes a space, about a two-inch space between boards and the tarpaper outside. That's all the insulation. And in the winter, [even] in March, the wind will howl through, and was it ever cold... we piled up about a dozen blankets, army blankets on us to keep us warm."

Miura, with her expertise in dermatology, noted the skin rashes arising from stress of the new and unfamiliar surroundings. "Here people are all scared, worried, and then a lot of things happen when they become worried.... They get different kinds of what we call neurodermatitis, from nerves and all that. Then sometimes they get stomach problems." There was, in fact, a high incidence of peptic ulcers, in addition to the high rates of psychoneurosis and hypertension within Manzanar.

"Well, you can't tell them not to worry, because you're in the same position, you don't know. Because you don't know what the outcome of the war's going to be at that time. It's just impossible to kind of counsel them, you have to console them, but you can't console them too well," observed Miura.

The two-room hospital was painfully inadequate, and new facilities were established in an entire 100-foot-by-20-foot barracks in April. There was room now for a pharmacy, laboratory, X-ray room, and ten-bed hospital. But this still was not enough. Ground was broken for a new, army-issue, 250-bed hospital, which would finally be opened in July.

Before the facility was completed, the small medical staff had to grapple with a serious procedure on May 16, 1942. Explained Miura: "... we had this one kid that got shot by the MP in the arm because he asked if he could go out and pick up a piece of wood so he could make a table [or a chair] for his mother. I don't know whether the MP understood or not, but when [the boy] started picking up the thing, he thought [the MP] said yes...He got shot in the elbow. So then we had to take that bullet out...We had to sterilize everything, gloves, everything in hot boiling water, and operate that way."

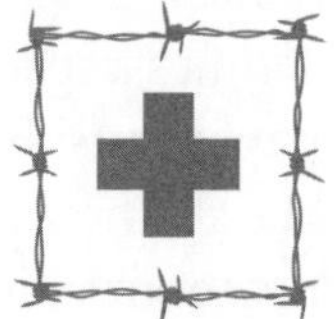

5. ESTABLISHING CAMP HOSPITALS

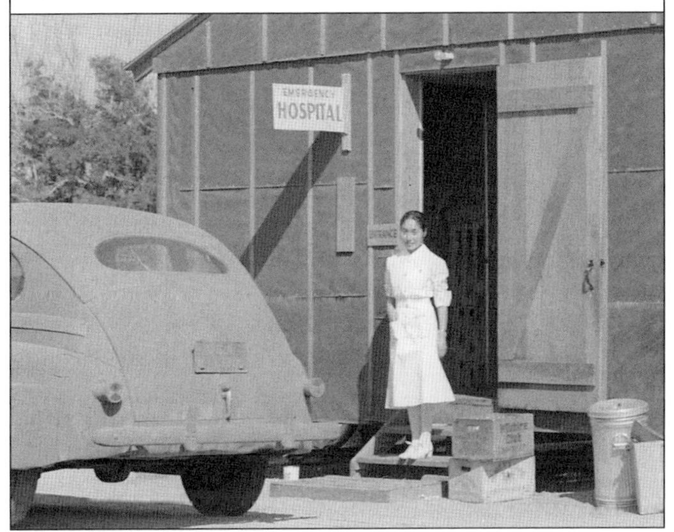

When our family arrived at Heart Mountain, Wyoming, my father found that the camp was not ready for habitation.

—Richard S. Kinoshita on his father Robert S. Kinoshita, MD

After spending at least two months in one of the temporary detention centers, Japanese Americans were then moved to permanent detention in Arizona, Arkansas, California, Colorado, Idaho, Oregon, Utah, Washington, and Wyoming. Among the first inmates to arrive were doctors and nurses, who were faced with the task of creating hospitals in barracks. In time, standalone buildings were constructed for hospital and operating rooms. Due to the lack of medical personnel during wartime, medical students often had to step in and assume the duties of full-fledged doctors.

SHIGERU HARA

From Arborga Assembly Center, Dr. Shigeru Hara and his wife were moved to Tule Lake Relocation Center in Northern California. By the time the Haras arrived, people from Washington and Oregon were already in place: "They were mostly farmers, small farmers. They were in charge of everything there."

But now, with the influx of approximately eight thousand large-scale farmers and urbanites from the Sacramento area, both the power and supervisory positions shifted to the Northern Californians. "It created a bad, bad feeling because all the managers were replaced. So when we got there, there were all these doctors there. The hospital was pretty busy, and they gave us one square block, all for medical personnel only, close to the hospital."

Here in Tule Lake, Hara was reunited with his Marquette classmate and friend Dr. Henry Sugiyama. The two had their medical degrees but not their licenses. The camp administration agreed to give them clearance to take their board examinations in Sacramento. "So they drove us down there in a car and left us with my wife's American friend, and we stayed there three days.

"We went down there, and Sugi used to say, 'There's a curfew.'

"I said, 'They don't know we're Japanese. They think we're Chinese.'

"But anyway, nothing happened. Nobody picked on us, and we passed the board exam and became doctors."

ROBERT S. KINOSHITA

Dr. Robert S. Kinoshita, who had spent the prior six years serving more than six thousand members of the Civilian Conservation Corps in rural areas in southern Oregon, was very familiar with working under primitive conditions. "When our family arrived at Heart Mountain, Wyoming, my father found that the camp was not ready for habitation," said Kinoshita's son Richard. "Dad would also be a WRA doctor at the camp. He was used to large installations, and it was apparent to him that this camp was not ready for people.

"They were assigned to Block 21, Barracks 6, Room D. There were mattresses. No beds to put them on. They slept on the floor. There was no stove. I don't know if you know it or not, but there were no locks on the doors, because the army had the right to inspect any time they wanted, and they did."

It was in Heart Mountain, according to son Richard, that Kinoshita began to have symptoms of gastrointestinal discomfort and bleeding stomach ulcers, which he self-diagnosed as signs of stress due to the incarceration. The Kinoshitas' second child, Richard, was due in October 1942. "My mother refused to let me [be] born in the camp," explained Richard. Evelyn Kinoshita was apparently concerned that the government might deny her child American citizenship. "She went to the camp director and said that I was going to be born in a real town, with a name, and not a bare patch of ground that somebody had put together and put barbed wire around. For whatever reason, that was allowed. Mother and Father were taken under armed guard in an army car, in the middle of the night, during a snowstorm, to Cody, Wyoming, where I was born. My mother said that they were treated very nicely by the staff. My father said that the attending physician was very apologetic for the fact that Dad obviously was qualified as a doctor. But Nisei doctors were not allowed to practice medicine [there] except for at the center, relocation center itself. So they had no standing anywhere else."

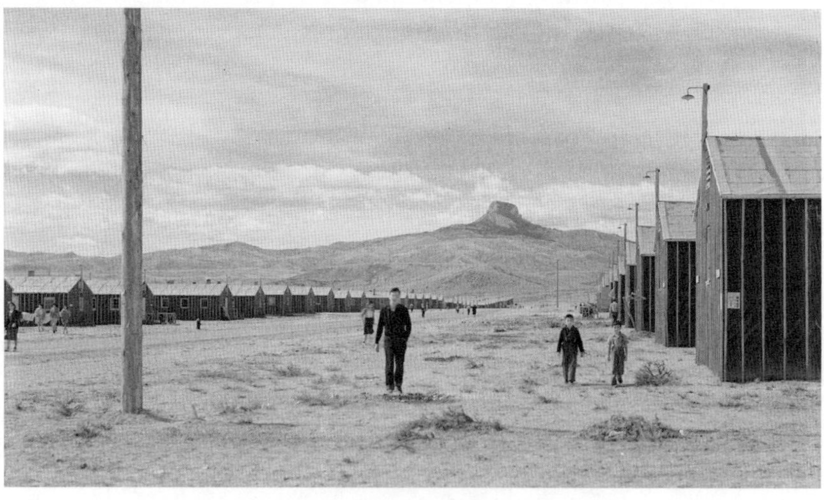

Heart Mountain Relocation Center, Wyoming.

FRANK CHUMAN
MASAKO (KUSAYANAGI) MIURA
MARY (SAKAGUCHI) ODA
YOSHIYE TOGASAKI
TOSHI YAMAMOTO

On June 1, 1942, the Manzanar Assembly Center was transferred from the jurisdiction of the army-controlled WCCA to the War Relocation Authority (WRA). The more permanent camp's name officially changed to the Manzanar Relocation Center. Under the WCCA, the doctors received $16 a month, the highest wages possible. When the WRA took over, they received a raise—to $19 a month. In contrast, physicians on the outside in private practice would average an annual income of $4,441.

With the opening of the new Manzanar Hospital on July 22, 1942, the medical staff now had 250 beds instead of a mere fourteen to accommodate patients. Their previous facility in Block 7 didn't have enough mattresses, and babies rested in cardboard boxes or makeshift cribs constructed from discarded lumber. But now, according to hospital administrator Frank Chuman, the government was prepared to supply Manzanar Hospital with any supplies and equipment from army supply depots. "The medical people in San Francisco, [were] given instruction that whatever Manzanar needed would receive high priority next to the ones in combat or out in the field.... when we ordered things, within a week or so, it was loaded on in San Francisco, came by rail down to Bishop, and then unloaded and came by trucks.... Inventory list that was twelve inches thick [had] every conceivable thing that we needed or had use for in the hospital."

As the hospital was planned according to a U.S. Army standard, there were no provisions, however, to meet certain specific needs of the elderly, women, and children. "Things like Kotex... those things, they obviously didn't have. Baby formula, they didn't have. They didn't have certain types of architectural design for ramps for elderly people to walk up."

All those items would be ordered separately from the procurement's head office from outside vendors. "But we got them," said

Chuman. Special diets also needed to be prepared for post-surgery and ailing patients. The mess hall in Block 28 worked in conjunction with dieticians to provide special food.

"The hospital was the biggest single operation in the whole camp, because it operated twenty-four hours," explained Chuman. Workers were hired for the extensive laundry and telephone switchboard operations. Inexperienced young women and men became nurse's aides, orderlies, and medical stenographers. Two European American nurses were instrumental in their training. "They set up a nurse's aide training program which attracted twenty, thirty people in each class, just tremendous interest in that. And then after [the students] got this prescribed basic training, information, test, and so forth, they were then capped with these little hats showing that they were certified nurse's aides. This was a great thing. I remember several young guys who were orderlies; we called them orderlies. A couple of them became doctors back east...."

Dr. Miura supervised the training of the medical stenographers. "I asked for a lot of the young girls who knew typing and shorthand, and then had them come in and take dictation from the doctors, different doctors. Every night I would correct the papers, correct the medical language. So that they got rather proficient in their medical terms, and then with typing it out, it made it a lot easier for everybody too."

Mary (Sakaguchi) Oda, whose medical school education at the University of California was interrupted by Executive Order 9066, benefited from the training led by these more experienced physicians. Oda and most of her other family members had come directly to Manzanar when it was a temporary detention center. Oda applied to work in the hospital. "They let me learn to draw blood and do histories and physicals, because that's the one thing doctors hate to do, is histories and physicals. So they taught us to do histories, and they gave us a crash course in physical diagnosis."

Dr. Tetsui Watanabe, serving as a radiologist at Manzanar, taught Oda how to examine patients, while Dr. Jiro Muramoto, a general practitioner from Sacramento, trained her to do her first spinal tap in camp.

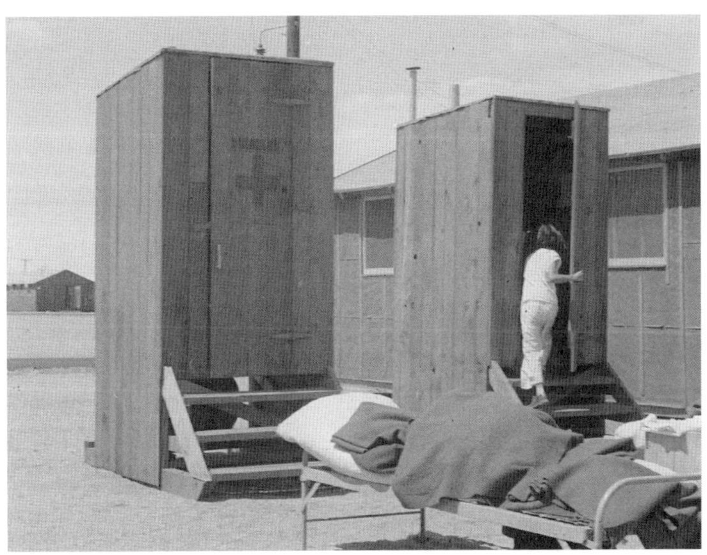

Manzanar Relocation Center, Manzanar, California. Hospital latrines for patients between the barracks, which served temporarily as wards.

"Goto was a wonderful surgeon... There were three nursing students that needed to complete six more months of training, so he somehow got their qualification, and he did a lot of lecturing. He was great.... all of us would go there and listen. He was a great lecturer, because he had to give the nurses enough didactic education so they could qualify and take... the nursing exam."

SHIGERU HARA
HENRY IWAO SUGIYAMA
MASAMICHI "MAC" SUZUKI

A twenty-passenger local bus took Henry Sugiyama and his family from Walerga Assembly Center to Tule Lake in May 1942. "We traveled all night to get to Tule Lake in the early morning," said Sugiyama. "And I didn't get a chance to unpack my bags for four days because I was working in the clinic. I was the first Japanese-speaking MD there. They had a Caucasian medical director, but he was of no use because the Japanese were all old people, and they spoke nothing but Japanese and very little English."

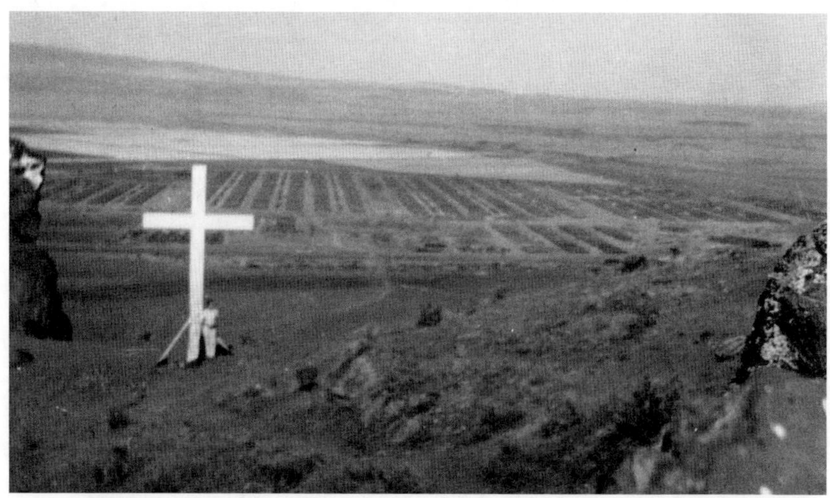

Overview of Tule Lake, with Dr. Henry Sugiyama standing next to cross.

In the beginning, Tule Lake, with the largest inmate population, had only fifty beds in its hospital. And like the other camp hospitals, it was not prepared to serve women and children. "We had to ask for all the medication for the kids, medication for the females, and medication for the babies, and the formula for the infants....

"It started to dribble in about two or three weeks later... because we made a screaming pitch at the medical director.

"'Hey, we need something more than something for an army hospital. And how about the X-ray?'

"'Well, it's coming. It's coming.'

"Well, it took how long before [the X-ray] machine came, four months."

After teaching Mary Oda the finer points of examining patients in Manzanar, Dr. Watanabe was transferred to Tule Lake because there were fewer doctors and no radiologists there. According to Suzuki, "Tets Watanabe was our radiologist, and he was an excellent radiologist. I learned a great deal from him."

Dr. George Hashiba, an Issei surgeon from Fresno, brought in his own personal equipment. "He brought a cystoscope, esophagus scope, and surgical tools," said Mac Suzuki. "He also performed neurosurgery, so he had his neurosurgical equipment.... He taught me how to use the cystoscope, and we had many patients. Many Issei had minimal medical care in the past. Hernia was a very common problem by the hundreds. They were using a truss. They came to the hospital for tonsillectomy, hemorrhoidectomy, and many non-acute type problems. We had a very busy clinic."

As Sugiyama checked on patients' blood pressure and pregnancies and treated diarrhea, vomiting, and colds, he carried an English-Japanese dictionary in one pocket and a Japanese-English dictionary on the other, because although he was exposed to some Japanese, he didn't speak it well. "There were times when days would go by before we could get some sleep." Even Hashiba, who was in his sixties, was making calls at three o'clock in the morning.

At times a specialist from the town of Tulelake or the University of Oregon was called and consulted. EKGs were printed out and even mailed. In one incident, Sugiyama even sent an EKG to his professor of internal medicine at Marquette.

The professor wrote back: "You're doing fine. Keep it up."

Suzuki worked under Dr. George Kambara, who was in charge of the Ear, Nose, and Throat (ENT) and ophthalmology clinic. The internees, according to Suzuki, had chronic tonsillitis with frequent sore throats. "Treatment was tonsillectomy. But we would do it under a local anesthesia. George Kambara had the training, so he taught me the operation. And we had many chronic sinus problems. I'd never heard of doing a sinus wash, but in those days, we took a big needle and insert [it] up the nose, and shove that needle right into the sinus area—then you flush it with…saline solution. I initially worried that the needle might go up into the brain, but apparently it never did."

Sacramento-born Kambara had graduated from Stanford University School of Medicine in 1941 and had entered an ENT residency at Stanford-Lane Hospitals in San Francisco. The Tule Lake Hospital and patients benefited directly from Kambara's experience and relationships cultivated with Stanford professors before the war. Kambara also showed Suzuki how to perform adult tonsillectomies. "After you remove [the tonsils], bleeders had to be tied," said Suzuki. "I can remember George teaching me how, by having an open can and placing a sponge there. You put your instrument in, and make a knot, which you slide it down to the bleeder, which is grasped and tied."

Shigeru Hara also witnessed how Kambara was able to receive help from his former alma mater. "He called his university, and they said, 'Set these cases aside, and we'll send a doctor there to help you.' So Stanford sent an eye doctor to help him to take care of these patients that he couldn't do.... The government won't take anything for nothing, so they gave [the Stanford doctor] one dollar."

Dr. Kazue Togasaki, the experienced obstetrician who had a practice in San Francisco before the war, taught Hara and his friend Sugi various techniques in how to deliver a baby, including the use of obstetrical forceps. The two young men had just completed a rotation in anesthesiology at Sacramento County Hospital. At that time, epidural anesthesia was virtually unheard of, so caudal anesthesia, in which the needle was inserted in the tailbone, was used. "I developed a technique that was entirely different from the schools. It used to work very well," explained Hara, who inserted the needle higher above the bone. He used this technique in the obstetrics department for deliveries supervised by Togasaki and Dr. George Baba, who was Togasaki's junior.

As Mac Suzuki had not yet completed his third and fourth years of medical school, he did not yet have much training in obstetrics. But through his work at the Tule Lake Hospital, he was able to assist Togasaki and even witnessed a Caesarian section. "It was a situation where the patient was having a difficult labor. Dr. Togasaki said [the] patient had a transverse arrest, where the baby's head is in transverse position. Head normally must be up and down, in order for delivery. Kielland forceps is used to rotate the baby's head; if delivery is not done correctly, one can tear the womb. Unfortunately this occurred but was immediately recognized by Dr. Togasaki. Patient was taken immediately to the operating suite, and a Caesarian section performed with resulting live infant. Mother did well post-operatively."

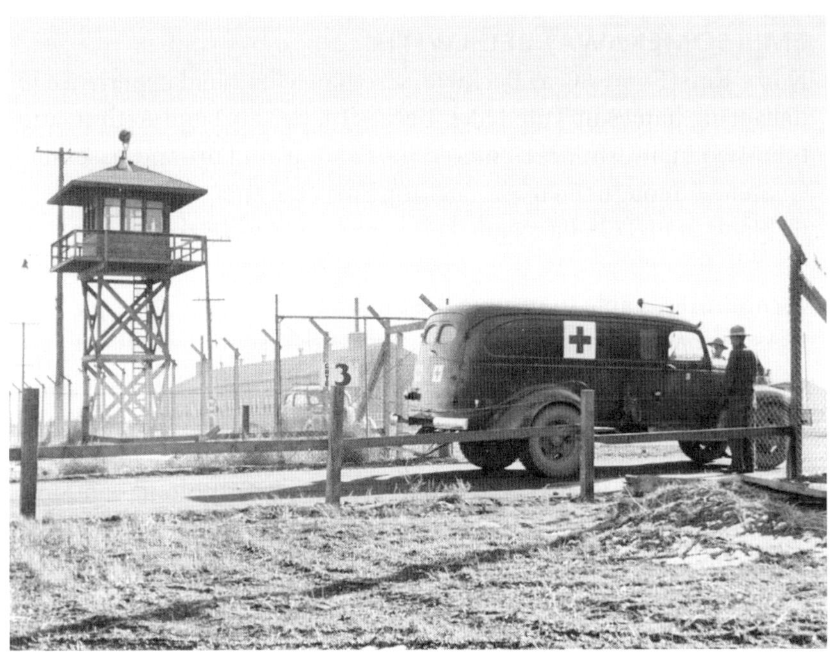

ABOVE: An ambulance stops at gate 3 Tule Lake Relocation Center.
BELOW: Women's ward in the temporary barracks hospital at Manzanar Relocation Center, Manzanar, California.

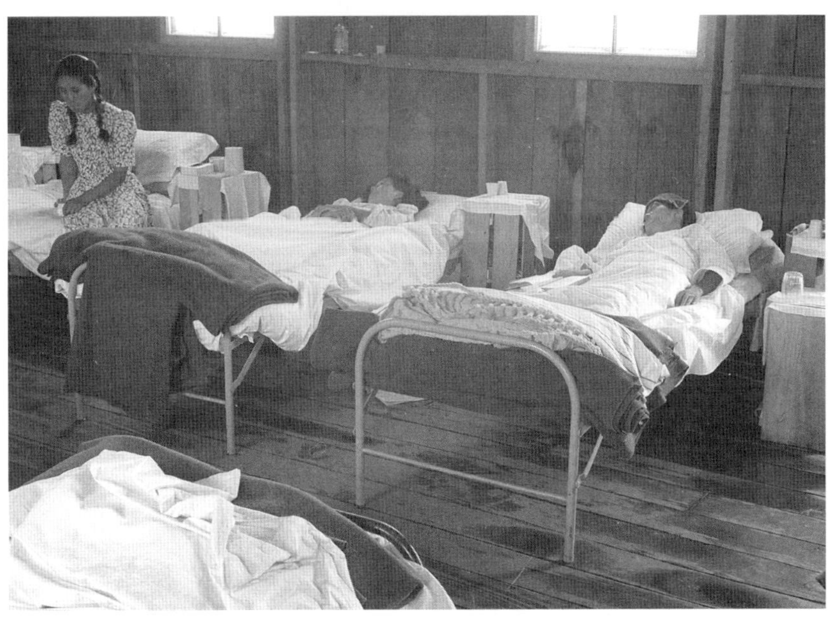

EMI (SOMEKAWA) BECKWITH

Nurse Emi (Somekawa) Beckwith also had a firsthand experience in delivering babies in Tule Lake. Beckwith, her husband Arthur, and their two infant children entered the camp from Portland Assembly Center in September 1942. Luckily, Emi's parents, the Yadas, were in Block 14 of Tule Lake, and the Somekawas were able to move to the adjoining block. With her parents agreeing to babysit their children, Emi was able to resume hospital work.

As she had previously indicated, Beckwith discovered that the Tule Lake Hospital was much more organized and better equipped than the makeshift medical clinic in Portland. There were special wards for maternity, surgery, and physical therapy. However, no provisions for blood transfusions were available. Supplies of blood were limited, and requests for certain blood types had to be ordered from the nearby town of Klamath Falls. In one case, an anemic patient started bleeding. As he had type "O" blood, he could not accept any other blood type, and was subsequently sent to the hospital in Klamath Falls. He subsequently survived his illness.

"We did have one pregnant lady who was a cardiac patient. She delivered finally, under oxygen," explained Beckwith. "We had the tent type of oxygen in those years. So we delivered her with the tent." The mother, unfortunately, died in childbirth, but the baby was born healthy.

Beckwith worked the 3:00 to 11:00 P.M. shift. Whenever it was time for a delivery, she would tell the ambulance driver, "You'd better go after any doctor on call."

"I'd usually get them on time," she said, "but once in a while you'd have a lady coming in, and they're ready to deliver right now. So I just delivered them. Then I'd have to make a report saying that so and so delivered. But then the doctor would come in the morning and check on them."

"In fact, when we were in Tule Lake, I think I must have delivered ten babies," concluded Beckwith.

ROBERT OBI

After assisting Drs. Shigekawa, Kuroiwa, and others at Santa Anita, Robert Obi was sent to Amache on the windswept plains in the southeastern corner of Colorado where he became chief X-ray technician for more than 7,300 detainees. "The X-ray technique was "very similar to what is used [in the early 1990s]," explained Obi. "Apparatus was not quite as complicated, but still it was very similar.... We did a lot of those orthopedic bone X-rays. We did GI [gastro-intestinal] studies. We did barium enemas. We did a lot of chest X-rays—took films."

Obi also saw simple medical cases in the clinic, such as skin rashes and colds. The most critical cases were transferred to outside hospitals in Denver. Also working in the Amache hospital was Dr. Benjamin Makoto Higashi, a Japan-born immigrant who moved to Honolulu in 1922 when he was nine. At the time, there were limited educational opportunities in Hawai'i so Higashi attended college on the mainland and received his MD from the College of Medical Evangelists at Loma Linda in 1939. He completed an internship and residency in 1942 at White Memorial Hospital in Los Angeles where he met his future wife, Dr. Lillian Shigemi Hamaoka. Married just four days before Pearl Harbor, the newlyweds ended up in Amache, where Benjamin served as head of surgery at age twenty-nine. During his three years there, Dr. Higashi performed more than five hundred operations and never lost a patient. Meanwhile, Lillian gave birth to their first child, Barbara, one of 415 babies delivered at Amache.

MASAMICHI "MAC" SUZUKI

With the overcrowded living situation in all ten camps, certain communicable diseases spread quickly. In Tule Lake, for example, Mac Suzuki recalled, "We had a very bad German measles epidemic during the first winter. We had a lot of sick children and babies. They were so sick. Some of them would be just covered in red with the rash. We didn't lose anyone though, fortunately, and the hospital just got filled up. So we went from barrack to barrack to find out if there were any children needing medical care. I can remember. I just tagged along

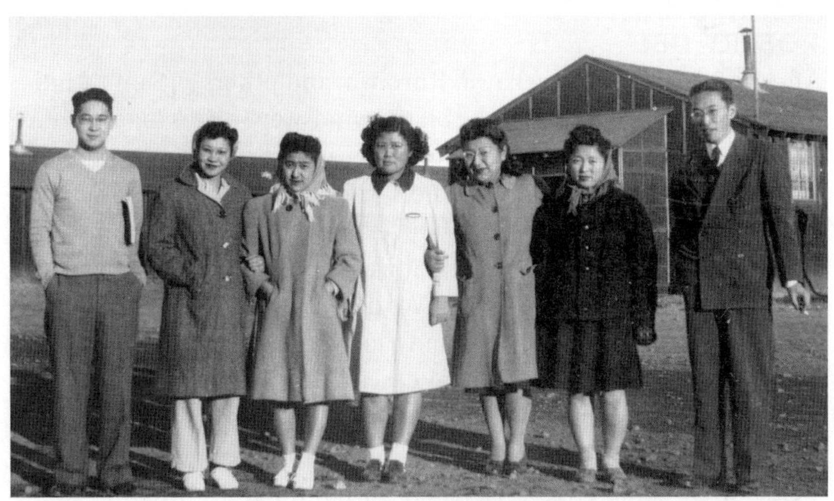

Dr. Masamichi "Mac" Suzuki (left), five nurse's aides, and
Dr. Henry Sugiyama (right) at Tule Lake.

with one of the family doctors. Several of them went in different jeeps, going through giving them proper treatment and medicine."

Not much could be prescribed for those diagnosed with German measles. Calamine lotion, of course, was dispensed for rash and itching. "You could give them some antipyretic for high fever. Not much you can do about it but bid for time. The unfortunate part is that German measles is generally a very mild measles, but when it occurs on adolescents it can get bad. So we had some very sick adolescents from German measles."

WILLIAM SATO

William Sato remembered a doctor, a professor of internal medicine in the Berkeley area, who was specializing in the study of valley fever, or coccidioidomycosis. Valley fever was a respiratory disease that was contracted by inhaling spore-laden dust. According to Sato, signs of valley fever had been seen in the Tulare Assembly Center. But it did not reach large numbers until inmates were moved to Arizona concentration camps in Gila River and Poston, where the fungal spores were endemic in the soil.

Tule lake WRA Camp

September 22, 1942

Dear Doctor Reichert, SURGERY PROF. STANFORD

Since leaving Stanford Lane Hospitals on March 26th I have been to Sacramento, my home town, to Marysville WCCA Concentration Camp, and finally to Tulelake WRA Project in Modoc County here in the upper corner of California. It has been a hectic experience and one that I would not like to repeat.

The hospital here in Tulelake is quite nice having eight wards each accommodating about 18 to 24 patients. There is one major operating room and one minor. There are 11 doctors and 2 medical students to run the place which averages about 100 patients. The out-patient department averages 400 daily. My Ear, Nose and Throat Clinic ranges betwee 37 and 62 patients daily.

Appendectomies are the most common operation done here. There was one gastroenterostomy, that being done by the open method. Since then I have talked one of the surgeons into wanting to try the aseptic technique of Martslov (spelling?) with those special clamps. We do not have access to various journals of the past, so I would like to know if you could list some references and places where we could obtain reprints as to the technique and results. We would also like to know where the Martslov or Wangensteen clamps fo/aseptic technique of gastric resection and anastomosis could be purchased and as to their cost.

We have one gastric resection waiting for action and the surgeon is anxious to try these new clamps, so we would appreciate your early answer on this matter.

I know Dr. Holman was quite sold on these clamps. I was very impressed too during my short stay on the surgical service.

I have heard that your staff is getting depleted by the call from the armed forces. I often wished I was back at Stanford finishing my residency in Ear, Nose and Throat.

Please extend my best regards to Drs. Dobson, King, Scarborough, and the others on the Surgical service. Also to John in charge of the surgical laboratory. Also to Dr. Holman wherever he may be.

Sincerely yours,

Letter to Dr. Reichert, Professor of Surgery at Stanford University, from Dr. George Kambara, September 22, 1942, describing his work in the hospital at Tule Lake.

"You know the desert is a very delicate thing," said Sato. "You only have a crust like that, and especially when they were building the camp, it was all broken down, and [the dust] was just fine. And every time, the wind blows it just carries it right up in the air."

One patient had been "several hundreds pounds, a big man," said Sato. "He was about the same age as I was. He caught it, and unfortunately, he didn't make it. There wasn't any particular therapy for it other than bed rest." Like tuberculosis, symptoms were cough, loss of appetite, and weight loss. There were apparently two types of coccidioidomycosis: a serious but self-limiting primary form and a severe progressive infection that spreads throughout the body and can be particularly lethal.

IWAO GEORGE KAWAKAMI

Iwao Kawakami, who had been accepted to Washington University Medical School in St. Louis, had worked as a medical statistician for a few months at the Gila River Hospital. On a plain piece of paper, he recorded admissions, discharges, and deaths, but did not note specific diseases. There he met a valley fever specialist who had also spent some time at the Santa Anita Assembly Center. "He showed me the Petri dishes, how they grew the [fungal spores], how overnight it grew up to the lid," said Kawakami.

Kawakami himself caught valley fever from the dusty camp conditions. "I had a... slight fever, and my knees swelled up on me," he said. In most cases, the spores affected patients' joints, with more severe cases permeating people's lungs and organs. Kawakami, on the other hand, experienced infection only in his knees. In terms of a treatment, there wasn't any. "It was just rest," said Kawakami. "They had no medication for it."

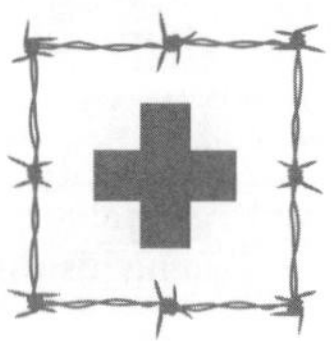

6. HELPING THE CAPTORS

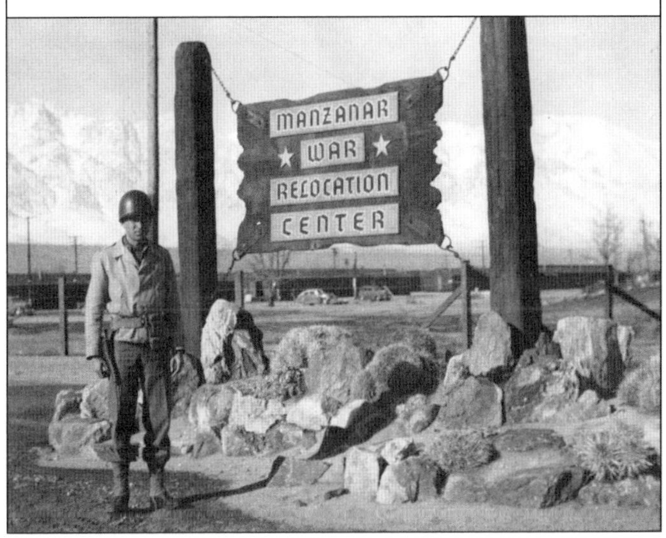

One of the shocking things was he described how they would pick him up from this camp and take him to the other side of the camp where he helped do induction physical to draftees.

—Augustus "Gus" Tanaka, MD, regarding his father Benjamin Masayoshi Tanaka, MD, during his captivity at Fort Sill alien internment camp

HOMER YASUI

From Pinedale, teenager Homer Yasui accompanied his mother and sister to Tule Lake and went to work as an orderly. "One day when I was on duty, they brought in this young white male who was severely burned. I don't know why they brought him to the Tule Lake Hospital. There we had a hospital that was built along army lines, but he was severely burned, mortally burned. He was from Merrill. Now Merrill is between the town of Tulelake, which is in California, and Klamath Falls was in fact about midway. So I don't know where this kid came from. But the story that we got later was that his car had stalled so I guess [as] it was common in those days, he took off the carburetor cap and poured a little bit of gasoline in there. He was looking at it when his friend stepped on the starter and that ignited the gasoline. It spewed the gasoline all over. He caught on fire, and he got severely burned.

"So they brought him to the Tule Lake Hospital. I don't, to this day, know where they brought him from, but if it was from Merrill, it would have been closer to go to Klamath Falls where there was a regular hospital. But anyway, they brought him to our hospital. In those days, we didn't have penicillin. The army had it. You know it was prioritized to the armed forces. [Silver nitrate was commonly used but] we didn't have any other treatment except... gentian violet. That's what the doctors [ordered] because [it] was kind of a weak antiseptic. We painted it. It's purple stuff, and we painted it. Of course, it smelled awful, you could smell his cooked flesh and all that.

"He hadn't completely lost consciousness, but after a day or so, you know every four hours the orderly's job was to paint the burn with more gentian violet. A few hours later, he was moaning and groaning, telling his folks, who were sitting there, sitting anxiously waiting, 'I don't want to be in this damned Jap hospital!'

"Oh man, here we're doing whatever we could for the guy. We didn't have much. We just had IV's you know, and he didn't want to be in a damned Jap hospital. He died. He died of his burns. But anyway, there wasn't much we could do."

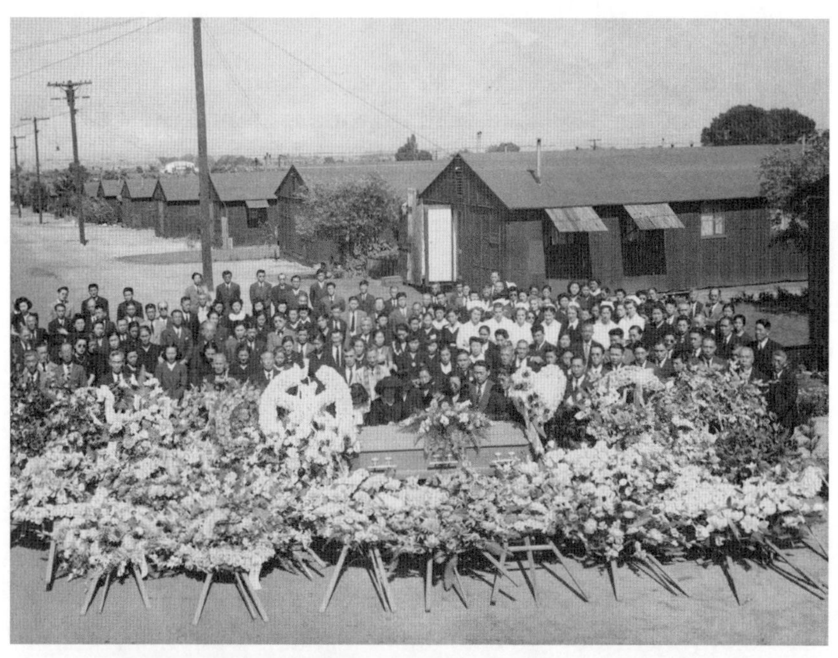

Above: A funeral at Manzanar Relocation Center. Below: A view of a Manzanar cemetery. Photos by Thelma McBride, JANM Collection.

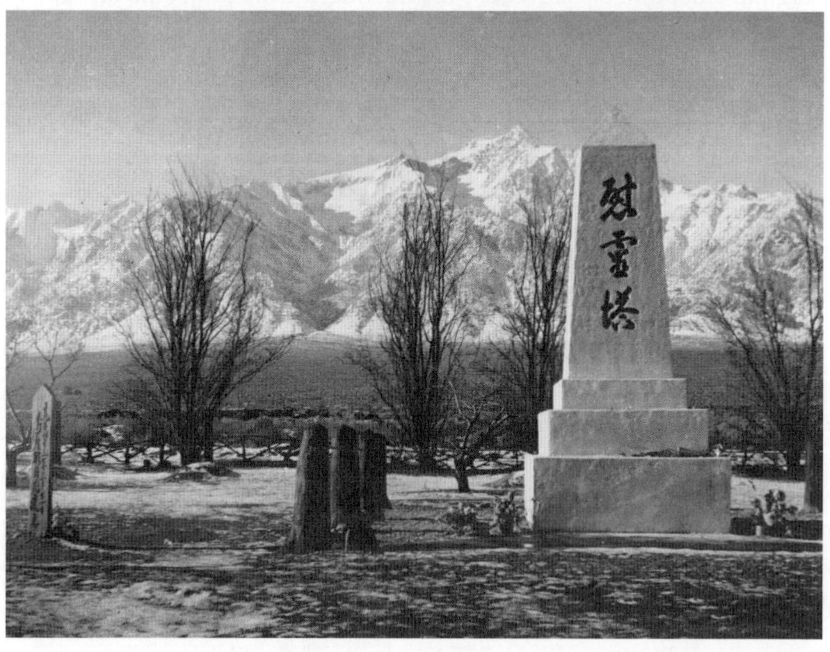

AUGUSTUS "GUS" TANAKA

Gus Tanaka, meanwhile, tried to stay in touch with his father, who was being moved from one alien internment camp to another. "I remember getting a letter from Dad, and the only thing was the date, and it said, 'Dear Gus.' The rest was all cut out and signed. The body of the letter was all gone.

"The censor had just cut everything out. They didn't block it out with black ink. They would just cut it out. Once in a while, they let some innocuous thing like 'how are you?' or 'I'll write again,' the rest of it was all cut out....

"My recollection was the next place... Fort Sill, Oklahoma, and that was a military installation. Apparently they used a section of this camp, maybe they used the stockade... but it was a barbed wire secured place. The thing that amazed me, after the severe censorship in Missoula, they let substantive information come through in the letters he wrote.

"One of the shocking things was he described how they would pick him up from this camp and take him to the other side of the camp where he helped do induction physicals to draftees....

"Because they didn't have enough doctors available to do the physicals. He pointed out the irony of all this."

SHIGERU HARA

As in all the other WRA hospitals, the doctors of Tule Lake were not allowed to treat the non-Japanese American staff workers. "I remember one time we had a heavy American lady teacher who had a bellyache," remembered Shigeru Hara. Dr. A.B. Carson, "who was the head of the [hospital], was the only person that could take care of the American people.... No Japanese doctor could touch American personnel.... That was the ruling then. He was a tuberculosis doctor, so he didn't know very much about surgery, I guess. But since he was the only American doctor, he had to operate on her. He asked me to give anesthesia for an appendectomy. So I gave anesthesia then. We used to do anesthesiology in the county hospital where our surgeons were young and very fast. They'd do appendectomies in about fifteen minutes. Well, this time I gave and gave and gave anesthesia for an hour and a half, and the doctor couldn't find the appendix.

"So finally he asked Dr. Harada, the Japanese surgeon, 'Could you help me?'

"So [Harada] said, 'Why sure.' So he went over there, put his fingers right in and pulled it right out."

It turned out that it was not the appendix at all, but a mittelschmerz, where the ovary had bled excessively during ovulation.

Hara remembered another case in which three, four European Americans drove into camp in a car. "We need a doctor right away because our friend got shot," they said.

"[The administration was] saying no Japanese doctor could look at American people, and they were arguing about it. So I went to look at it, and the man was already dead."

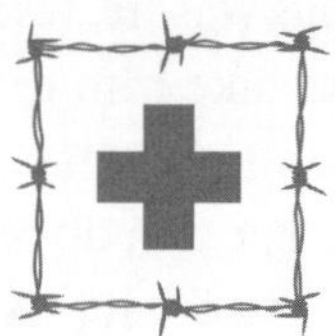

7. A TIME TO IMPROVISE

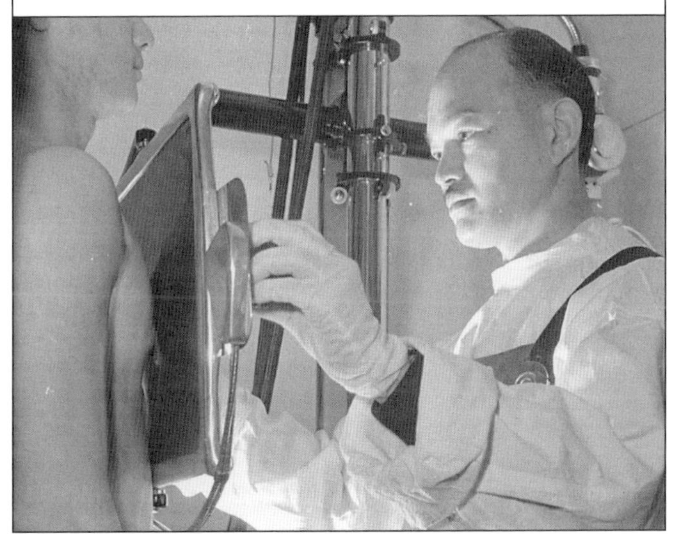

So they gave us the hand drill.
We cleaned it all up and sterilized it,
and the doctor used it.

—Shigeru Hara, MD, in Tule Lake Relocation Center

Y. FRED FUJIKAWA

During Dr. Fred Fujikawa's experience on Terminal Island before the war, "the most exciting thing that happened in my practice of medicine was the introduction of antibiotics on a therapeutic basis. It was around the latter part of the 1930s that the first sulfa medication was introduced."

Penicillin came towards the end of World War II, but was still not widely available to the general public and not in camp. As a result, Fujikawa turned to sulfa medication to treat a girl who had a ruptured appendix. "We opened her up, and her abdomen was just full of pus. We irrigated her as well as we could and sprinkled some sulfathiazole crystals all over her belly and inside of her belly," said Fujikawa.

The procedure was a success. Decades later, in the 1980s, Fujikawa would meet his former patient, who was still very much alive.

SHIGERU HARA

According to Jensen (1999), tuberculosis was the third leading cause of deaths of internees one year of age or older. The containment and treatment of tuberculosis were a challenge in light of the crowded living conditions and the Japanese community's fear of the disease. While Poston reported 153 cases of tuberculosis, Tule Lake had only ten on record. Yet Shigeru Hara, who had tuberculosis as a child, remembers when some tubercular patients were sent to Tule Lake Hospital from the Monterey area of California. According to Hara, these patients filled two hospital wards. "Some of them were in real bad shape, because you know Japanese hate tuberculosis like leprosy. If they found a tuberculosis case in the block, everybody wants to move out," said Hara. As a result, patients with severe cases of tuberculosis were usually taken out of camp and isolated in certain outside hospitals.

According to Hara, Tule Lake Hospital was in a good position to treat the tubercular patients. "The nurse in charge of it was a very good nurse, and she was a University of California graduate," he said. "She took very good care of them, and that's when we found that we had to do pneumothorax [therapeutic measure to collapse the lung]."

Hara, in fact, had some experience in administering pneumothorax at the county hospital before the war. In Tule Lake, Shigeru had no fears about working with the TB patients. "I had tuberculosis myself, so why should I worry about it? But the other doctors, the older doctors, they didn't care to go to the tuberculosis ward, especially the surgeons."

"They looked for a machine, and they didn't have any gadgets to use it. So I got some of those one one-liter bottles, IV bottles, got two of them and put some tubes on it and built a gadget to shove the air into the chest. I just made it; it was very simple. We used that all the time I was there."

Ironically, Hara later heard that a pneumothorax machine was discovered in a supply room. Nobody had apparently known what it was.

Hara and his colleagues improvised another procedure, this time involving treatment of a man's broken hip. It all began, explained Hara, when some Issei in Tule Lake sent for *koji*, malted rice yeast, from Denver. "The guards didn't know anything. They just looked at it and said, 'It's rice. I don't know why these guys are buying more rice from [the] outside.'" But this was used to make sake, or rice wine. "So one winter, one of the fellows, I guess an old man, drank too much and so he was sliding down the hill on cardboard or something, and his foot struck against a stump...and it broke his hip. He was brought into the hospital, and Dr. [George] Hashiba, who was a very excellent surgeon...looked at him, and he said, 'We need a drill.' There were no drills in the surgical supply. So we went to the garage and asked them to loan us a drill. The man said, 'Well, we can't send it out, but if it's to save a man's life, you can have it.'

"So they gave us the hand drill. We cleaned it all up and sterilized it, and the doctor used it. And he fixed the man's hip."

MASAMICHI "MAC" SUZUKI

Mac Suzuki was impressed with the older doctors in Tule Lake. "I got good training, a training that I never would have gotten in the medical field while I was at camp. I was fortunate enough to be in a camp where we had very good doctors, like Dr. Hashiba, who

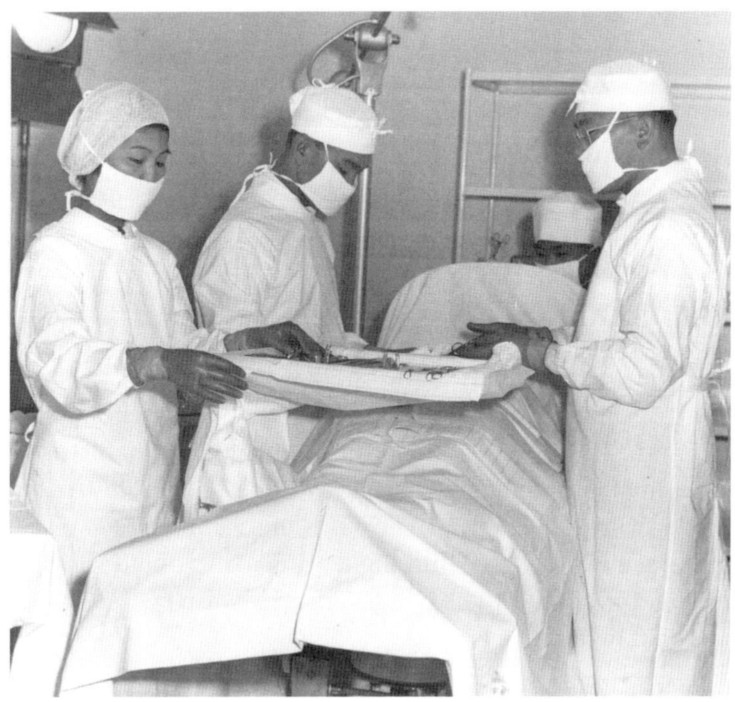

Santa Anita Detention Center Hospital c. 1942 (summer). Staff of doctors operating on a patient. LEFT TO RIGHT: Dorothy Kobata (nurse), Dr. Fred Fujikawa, Dr. Sakaye Shigekawa, Dr. Thomas Abe. Dr. Shigekawa is giving anesthesia to patient.

was enthusiastic, always plugging the younger doctors to do better. Teaching us and really instilling in us the nicety of practicing medicine."

Suzuki described Hashiba as "a very fascinating individual because his whole life revolved around medicine." An Issei trained at Stanford Medical School, Hashiba had been a surgeon at Fresno County General Hospital and sometimes used his skill to do complicated procedures in camp. "There was a child who'd developed encephalitis," explained Suzuki. "In order to relieve the pressure on the brain, he decided he'd make a trephine, you know, make a hole in the [skull]. Then, I remember putting a needle in to drain the brain, but I think that was about the only [brain procedure done while I was in camp]."

According to Suzuki, Hashiba would use his vacations before the war to visit various medical facilities. One time he dissected a cadaver at Stanford in the anatomy laboratory. Other times he went to various clinics on the East Coast. "What did you learn?" Suzuki asked Hashiba.

"I learned if the doctors there can do it, I can do it!"

MASAKO KUSAYANAGI MIURA

Before the war, Dr. Masako Kusayanagi Miura had studied syphilology and other venereal diseases during her residency at Los Angeles County General Hospital, but she saw few cases in camp. "... but there was one case [at Manzanar] where this fellow had general paresis of the brain. They go wacky, and they didn't know what to do with him. So then I thought, *Well, we used to give malarial treatment for the fever, fever therapy.... The only thing I have here to give him fever is typhoid.* So I gave him higher doses of typhoid shots, kept increasing the dose until he had fever.... He wasn't cured, but then he was a lot better."

BENJAMIN MASAYOSHI TANAKA

Dr. Benjamin Tanaka had been transferred from one Immigration and Naturalization Service detention camp to another. He spent the last of his imprisonment in Santa Fe alien detention camp in New Mexico, where he served as chief physician. Several Caucasian doctors were actually officially in charge of the medical facilities, but they would "just sign a bunch of papers and walk out. But they were the ones that got paid for supervising. In the beginning, they said they checked it out, but after a while, they had confidence in the work that... the prisoner doctors were doing, so they just signed off and endorsed the records. They were rarely seen actually," said Tanaka's son Gus.

One of the staff nurses was Nadine Benoit, who described to Gus his father's dedication. "Nadine would say how he would stick with his patients day and night, struggling to keep some of these patients alive when he didn't have all the equipment or the medications that he would say he'd like to have, and have no access to."

The hospital at the Santa Fe alien internment camp did not have

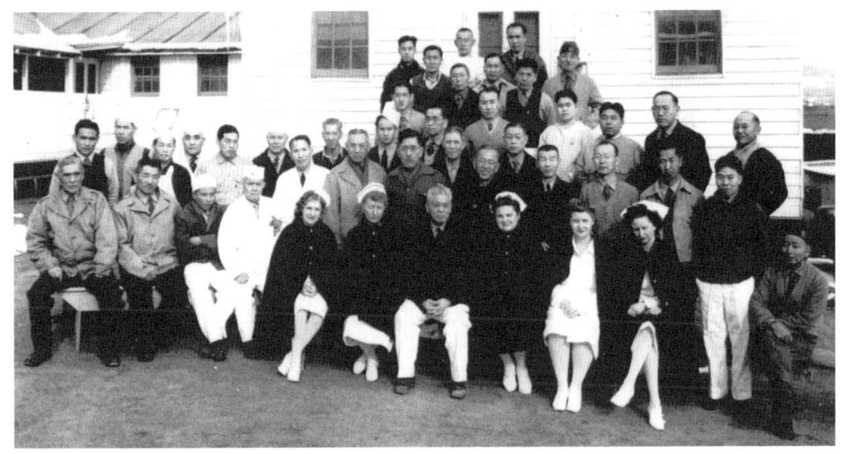

ABOVE: Santa Fe medical staff, Dr. Benjamin M. Tanaka, front and center, surrounded by nurses. To his left is Public Health Nurse Nadine Benoit, without her cap. BELOW: Signatures of Santa Fe medical staff. Photos courtesy of Dr. Gus Tanaka.

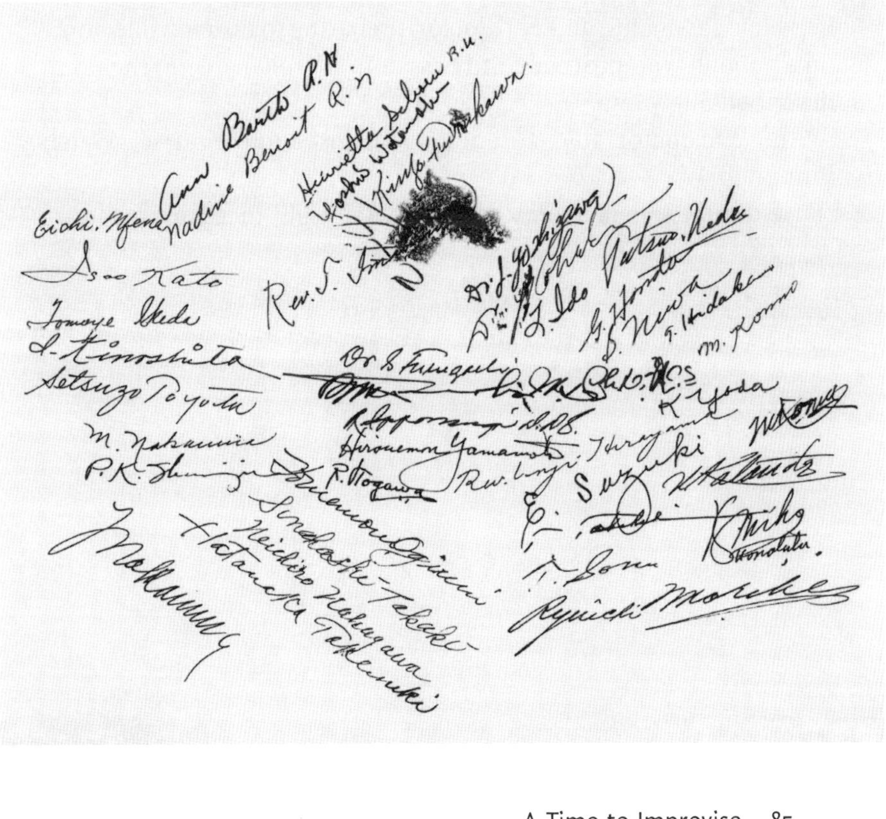

a formal operating room or high-functioning lights. "They're usually high intensity, high beam lamps so that it illuminates the field well," explained Gus. "But they had some cheap lamps that were not strong enough light, so... Nadine... described such things as Dad improvising reflectors using aluminum foil to throw the light back onto the field and so forth. She mentioned improvising retractors and other surgical instruments out of common things because the government did not supply all the equipment that they thought they needed. Little attachments to examining tables were devised by Dad and other people that were more mechanically talented, to make the things according to the way Dad would want it."

HENRY IWAO SUGIYAMA

At the Tule Lake Hospital, doctors were doing an average of six tonsillectomies in an hour. Henry Iwao Sugiyama witnessed one of his Berkeley classmates, an ENT doctor, preparing to do a tonsillectomy on a patient, who proceeded to pass out. "So the man's on the floor," described Sugiyama.

"And [the doctor] told the anesthesiologist and the nurse, 'Watch him.'

"He did the tonsillectomy. He finished it right there on the floor."

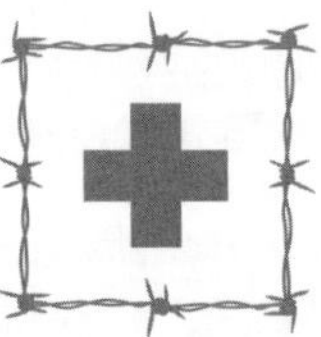

8. CAMARADERIE, RIVALRIES, AND CONFLICT

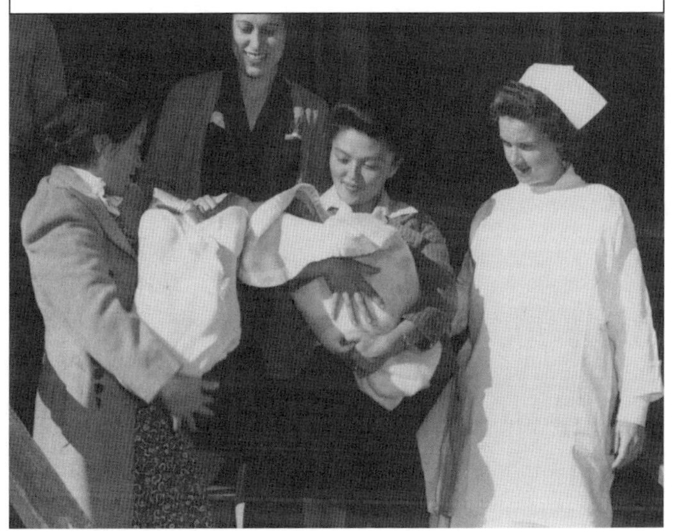

You didn't want to be on [a particular] *side, but there were times, when you felt one for him and one for her.*

—Toshi Yamamoto, regarding the relationship between Dr. James Goto and Dr. Yoshiye Togasaki in Manzanar

TOSHI YAMAMOTO

With Dr. James Goto's specialty in surgery and Dr. Yoshiye Togasaki's expertise in public health, tension was bound to erupt between these two strong personalities. Toshi Yamamoto was among those who witnessed arguments.

"So she said, 'Jim, you're wrong!'

"Then he would say, 'Togi, what makes you think you're right all the time?'

"It was embarrassing.... You didn't want to be on [a particular] side, but there were times when you felt one for him and one for her."

A more humorous subject of dissension was the use of the hospital refrigerator, which was meant for medicine, but was instead filled with high-quality Roquefort cheese and salami from Goto's brother. "Togasaki and he would go round and round and round, and he was going to fire all the girls that had anything to do with eating his cheese or salami. It so happened that all the girls who were undergraduates that were filling out their term had eaten a piece of it. He was going to fire them all," recalled Yamamoto.

"So I stepped in, and I said, 'I'm the one that gave everybody a piece of it, so fire me!'"

"I don't know why, but I got nothing but respect. Nothing but respect.

"And he looked at me, and he said, 'Well, if you say you gave them a piece, all right, but I'm not going to let them go through my cheese.'"

Yet Togasaki insisted that the refrigerator be reserved only for medical use. "She told Dr. Goto, 'Jim, I'm coming tonight, and I'm cleaning out the refrigerator. If there's anything in there that belongs to you, you'd better take it out before I get there.' And it was done, it was done."

MASAMICHI (MAC) SUZUKI

Since Mac Suzuki had some pathology experience at the University of California Medical School, he was called upon to conduct autopsies on people who died in camp. He would send tests to an outside doctor, who would subsequently return a report to the Tule Lake

Hospital. What Suzuki never imagined was that the autopsy room would one day play a role in preparing a pig for a pork roast.

"We were able to raise our own guinea pigs or rabbits for pregnancy tests," said Suzuki. "So we had a fellow who took care of raising these animals. We found out that we could get a pig, a big pig. I don't know whether we paid or whether the farm donated it but decided the hospital will have a barbecue. We get this great big fat pig and take it to the autopsy room, which had a concrete floor.

"We said, 'How are we going to kill this creature?' We want to be as humane as possible. I think ordinarily they cut their throat or slug a hammer over the head, I don't know exactly how the butchers did it. But we were going to be humane, we etherized it. So we poured ether, and finally the pig goes to heaven.

"Anyway the pig dies, and we had the kitchen roast it. Meanwhile we sold tickets. I can't remember, it was a few dollars. Here's the banquet night everything's ready. I don't remember how many tickets we sold. But finally the pork roast was served, and you know what?...A pig has a lot of fat, and the ether was absorbed by the fat. Pork roast was reeking of ether. We had a hilarious time. What a disaster!"

Deterred by the smell, the doctors didn't even taste the pig. The roast was thrown away and most of the money returned. "Maybe they decided a few dollars, they'd donate it to the hospital. But we didn't have our barbecued pork dinner."

Y. FRED FUJIKAWA

The doctors at Jerome Relocation Center in faraway Arkansas worked well together, according to Dr. Fred Fujikawa. "In camp, we got along fine. We worked hard. Treated the patients to the best of our ability, but we were short-handed in some respects. Equipment and supplies were of concern."

"And we had bull sessions, of course. And we grumbled about it. We'd say, 'When that [WRA head] Dillon Myer comes, we'll tell him off.'...Well, Dillon Myer finally did come, and he wanted to know how things were in the hospital and so forth. We sat around in a big circle and he said, 'Does anyone have anything to say? Any questions?'

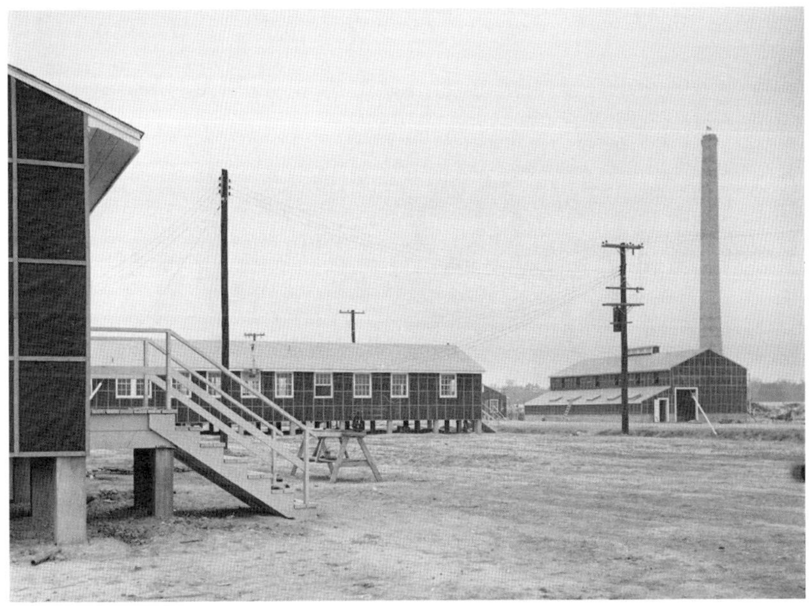

Jerome Relocation Center, Denson, Arkansas.

"No one said a word. So I started in and I told him...everything that we had been talking about.

"'You tell me, Doctor,' he said, 'You sound very bitter. I suggest you leave camp as soon as you can.'

"So I said, 'Okay. I will.'"

With that Fujikawa perused the bulletin board at the hospital. Seeing an opening at the Missouri State Sanatorium, Fujikawa decided that the next home for himself, his wife Alice, and their year-old son Denson Gen, would be near the small town of Mount Vernon, Missouri. While Fujikawa received a warm reception within the walls of the sanatorium, the townspeople of Mount Vernon apparently didn't feel the same way. "They weren't against me at all in the sanatorium, but some local people started agitating in the town of Mount Vernon, which was a mile away. The medical director came and told us to be careful."

A state representative, J.A. Gray, even supported an amendment preventing non-Missouri physicians from working in the state. "This doctor may be skillful, by the eternal gods, a Jap is a Jap," testified

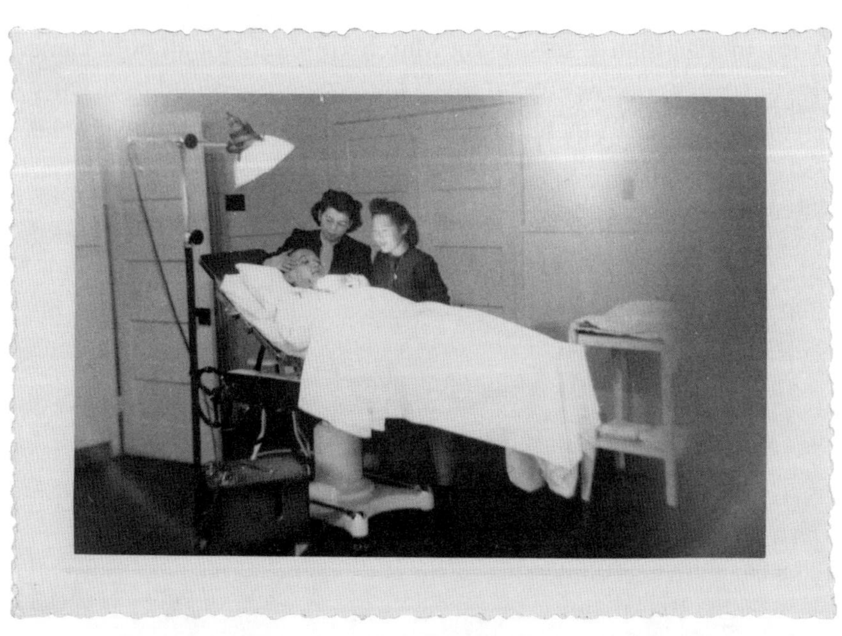

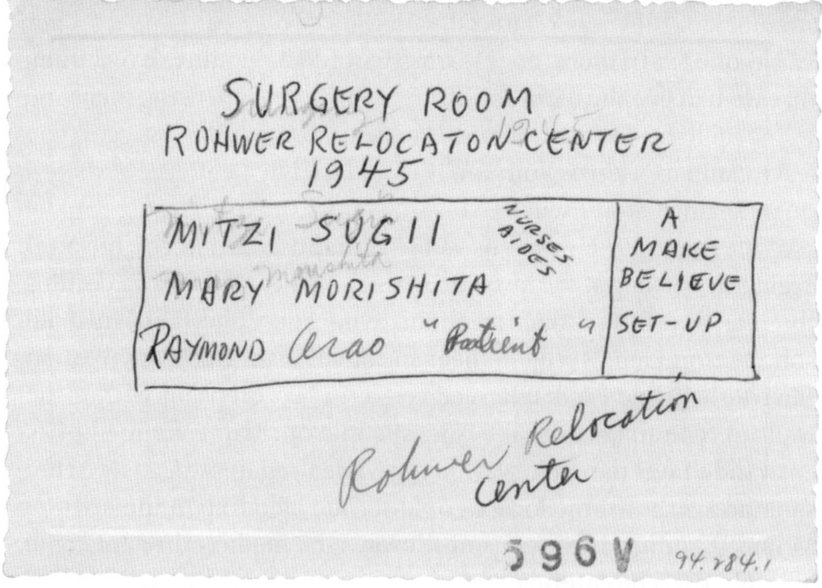

Interior of a surgery room at Rohwer Relocation Center, 1945. According to the inscription, this scene was a "make believe setup". Nurses aides are Mitzi Sugii and Mary Morishita. Raymond Arao is the patient. Two women look down at a patient who has a white cloth pulled up to his chest.

Gray in a legislative session on March 31, 1944. Not all politicians felt the same way. Representative O.K. Armstrong stood in defense of Fujikawa. "Why penalize this man who was born as much as an American as I, except that he has the blood of a different race in his veins?" he said. "This measure is aimed only at this one race. But we might be starting something here we can't stop. Regardless of intolerance elsewhere, we're not going to stand for it here in Missouri." The amendment failed to pass the legislature. Fujikawa continued his work alongside five other doctors in caring for six hundred patients, 70 percent of whom had tuberculosis.

SHIGERU HARA
MASAMICHI "MAC" SUZUKI

The chief medical officer during the early years of Tule Lake Hospital was Dr. A. B. Carson. "Carson was a director who just went along with everything that we did," remembered Suzuki, whose strongest memory of him was related to Carson's two Great Danes. "They came in, both of them, one time with porcupine quills all over their faces and inside the mouths. So, I remember anesthetizing them and then [pulling] out the quills."

On January 15, 1943, Carson was replaced by Dr. Reece Pedicord, an autocratic administrator who aroused the ire of many of the older physicians of Tule Lake. Shigeru Hara, then a young intern, however, had little problem with the controversial medical director. According to Hara, many operations were occurring at the Tule Lake hospital. "The doctors said, 'Well, all the people [who] are going out of camp have to be in excellent physical condition so they won't be a load on the community where they go.' So even a chronic thing like hernias and things like that—[which] people used to put up with, they operated on all of those things before they left." Hara himself participated in doing surgical procedures, such as phrenic nerve crush, a surgical treatment for tuberculosis common before the introduction of antibiotics.

Pedicord, on the other hand, apparently felt that there were too many surgeries being held at Tule Lake. "He used to say, 'Any case that has to be operated, you've got to let me see it first.' So some of those were acute appendicitis. By the time he got to see them, he made it pretty late and made it much worse. So that's why a lot of people were against him. But nobody lost their life because of it."

Hara, who volunteered for military service before he could be drafted as a "buck private," finally left camp in 1943. Wearing a uniform purchased in Medford, Oregon, Hara left Tule Lake as a first lieutenant in the U.S. Army. "All the soldiers were saluting me, [even] the guards. So all the girls in the hospital, they were really happy to see it."

Later on, Pedicord sent Hara a check for his overtime hours at Tule Lake. "I was shocked when I saw that," said Hara. He had good thoughts about his former employer, but days at Tule Lake were numbered for Pedicord.

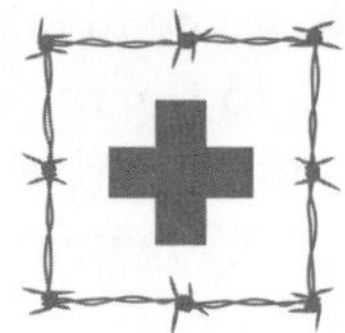

9. RIOTS AND SEGREGATION

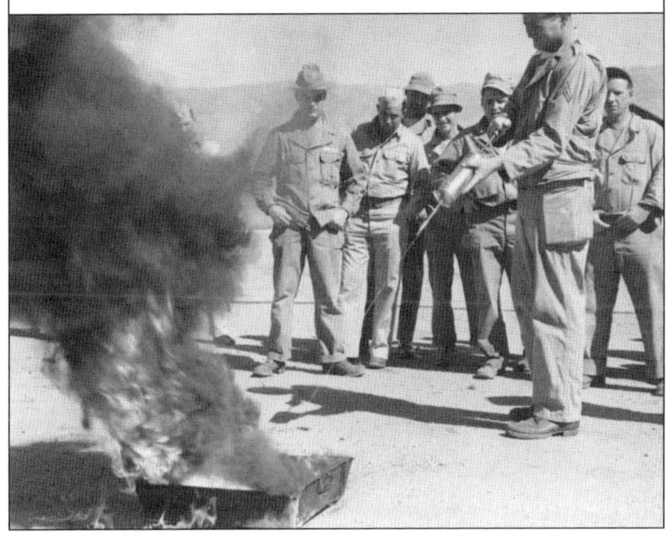

And as I got closer to the hospital area, I noticed that there was a line of soldiers with their helmets and the guns and bayonets.

—Masamichi "Mac" Suzuki, MD, regarding the events at Tule Lake on November 1, 1943

FRANK CHUMAN
MASAKO (KUSAYANAGI) MIURA

On December 6, 1942, violence broke out at Manzanar. A day earlier, a former Los Angeles restaurateur and Japanese American Citizens League leader, Fred Tayama, was severely beaten in his barracks by masked men. Camp administrators who saw him as a collaborator thought a popular Kibei mess hall leader, Harry Y. Ueno, was responsible and took him into custody and placed him in a county jail in the nearby town of Independence. His supporters, numbering from two to four thousand, protested the arrest, and fifty to seventy-five of them even went into the hospital in pursuit of Tayama, who was recuperating there from his injuries.

"A little nurse was standing by, and she said, 'No, you can't [go in] there,'" remembered Dr. Masako (Kusayanagi) Miura. The men told the nurse and the other medical staff to move out of their way.

"They said, 'No.'

"[The men] just pushed them aside and walked through all the wards, in and out, in and out. They went into the storage area, too, where we kept all our storage...supplies, and they couldn't find anybody. So they came out.

"They said, 'Well, let's get after Goto because he might have hid him or something.'

"So I said, '...come Jim, let's put on our pea coats and join the crowd.'...

"We went into the crowd and they never found us." Or Fred Tayama, who had safely hidden himself underneath an orthopedic bed.

Yet the conflict was not over. Later that evening, approximately five hundred men and boys gathered around the Manzanar jail to where Ueno had been moved. In spite of the detachment of military police, the crowd refused to disperse. Tear gas was released, and a driverless car was launched towards the police station. As the crowd scattered, the military police fired shots. One seventeen-year-old boy, James Ito, was killed instantly. Eleven others were injured.

Manzanar Hospital was transformed into an emergency room and trauma center. Dr. Goto, surgical nurse Yone Akita, and others worked feverishly to repair the bodies pierced by bullet wounds. Ten of them survived, but Jim Kanagawa, a twenty-one-year-old whose pancreas and stomach were perforated, died on December 11 from complications related to bronchial pneumonia.

The Ninth Service Command ordered a military inquiry in which Dr. Goto and other medical personnel were questioned. Manzanar Hospital administrator Frank Chuman remembered speaking with Dr. Goto at the time: "He talked to me after he was interrogated. And he said, 'The witnesses, and the nurses, the doctors, and particularly me were told to say that they were shot in the front, that the bullet wounds were in the front. Because I'm the one that did the surgery, I'm the one that knew where the bullet wound [entered, and] I refused to say they were shot in the front. I said they were shot either in the side or the back.' And he was quite adamant about that, and that got the military inquiry really upset, because he didn't change his story or his version of what he knew."

As a result, according to Chuman, Goto "was ordered summarily, just given a couple of hours, to get out. So he had to leave the hospital. . . ."

Drs. Goto and his wife, Miura, who was eight-months pregnant, left Manzanar for Topaz Relocation Center. During the train ride to Utah, Miura's feet began to swell. "I thought, 'Well, I've got to see a doctor when I get to Topaz.' I went out there, and all the Japanese doctors wouldn't see anybody, [they] wouldn't see me. . . . They were on strike. They wouldn't see us.'"

Hearing of Dr. Goto's mercurial personality and the "incident" at Manzanar, the medical staff was opposed to the couple joining their hospital. But that didn't change the fact that Dr. Miura needed medical attention. "I think I have a right to go outside and have somebody else treat me outside, since there's no one here to take care of me," she said at the time. She was granted permission from the Topaz medical director to go to Salt Lake City and see Dr. Ed Hashimoto, her former dentist's nephew. She eventually gave birth to a daughter, Denise, in February 1943. The two of them returned to Topaz, where Miura resumed work at the hospital. At first the head nurse expected Miura to pay for a babysitter out of her $19 monthly salary:

"Well, you can hire somebody and pay them the $12," the nurse said.

"Me work for seven dollars?" Miura replied. "No, I'd rather stay home with the baby than just work for seven dollars.... Unless you can come up with something better, I'm not going to work."

The hospital administration relented, and assigned a distant relative of Miura, Sei Ichioka, to take care of the baby. In time, the rest of the staff softened their hardline approach to Goto and Miura, who began training the young doctors in Topaz. The patients were very thankful, showing their appreciation to Miura with their gifts of artwork made from shells found at the foot of Topaz Mountain.

Meanwhile, it took two to replace Goto at Manzanar. Dr. Wilfred Yoichi Hanaoka, who earlier had been assigned to Heart Mountain Relocation Center, was moved to Manzanar to take over surgery, and Dr. Morris Little, a physician from Nevada, arrived to serve as the new chief of the medical staff. Little was not well received, and virtually ignored by the other hospital personnel, according to various accounts.

"The problem was the doctors already there didn't respect him and didn't pay attention to him," said Chuman. "The time that he came in... to the time I left in September '43, I never talked to him. He didn't talk to me. I didn't give a damn. I really didn't give a damn."

MASAMICHI "MAC" SUZUKI
YOSHIYE TOGASAKI

Dr. Yoshiye Togasaki had her share of health problems in her young life. Her left cornea had been so scarred due to a childhood illness that she could not use her left eye at all for practical vision. Then in September 1942, she suffered from uterine bleeding. "I think it was nothing more than overwork that started it. At that point they figured that my sister [Dr. Kazue Togasaki] didn't want to worry about me in Tule Lake while I was in Manzanar, so finally as soon as they could move me, they sent me to Tule Lake."

As no one at Tule Lake could clearly diagnose why she was experiencing so much bleeding, Togasaki requested that she be allowed to go to Children's Hospital in San Francisco. The WRA authorities finally agreed, as long as Togasaki paid for her own transportation as well as the services of a guard. "There I had a complete [workup], and at that time, they weren't sure what it was all about," said Togasaki. She eventually returned to Tule Lake, where the surgeon and her sister determined that a hysterectomy was in order. Five days after the surgery, Togasaki was back at work in the hospital working with pediatric patients. "That was in late October when I went to Tule then to San Francisco just about the Christmas holidays. I got back to Tule Lake just before the new year."

In January 1943, all ten permanent camps were to be engulfed in a political maelstrom over the government's institution of a so-called loyalty review program. As part of the program, each internee over seven years of age had to answer a questionnaire with two highly-charged "loyalty questions."

No. 27 was "Are you willing to serve in the armed forces of the United States on combat duty, wherever ordered?" No. 28 was "Will you swear unqualified allegiance to the United States of America and faithfully defend the United States from any attack by foreign or domestic forces, and forswear any form of allegiance or obedience to the Japanese emperor, or any other foreign government, power or organization?"

"The questionnaire was a big problem, and the wording of it created that problem," explained Togasaki. "We were there at the time the questionnaires were being answered and the emotions were as high as anything I had seen. [There were] those who believed that everyone should answer. They felt that we should be loyal enough and answer as much as we could. The other group felt that the government had no business asking the questions when we were there under duress without consent and that our citizenship rights had been abrogated. A very small number of this group were still loyal to Japan but primarily because they didn't dare be separate from their parents who were non-citizens. It is amazing that the complexity of this sort did not occur to the government."

The two Togasaki sisters stayed in Tule Lake until March 1943. "Then at that time," said Yoshiye, "the medical director said that the Togasaki sisters are too disruptive to this camp and he sent us all

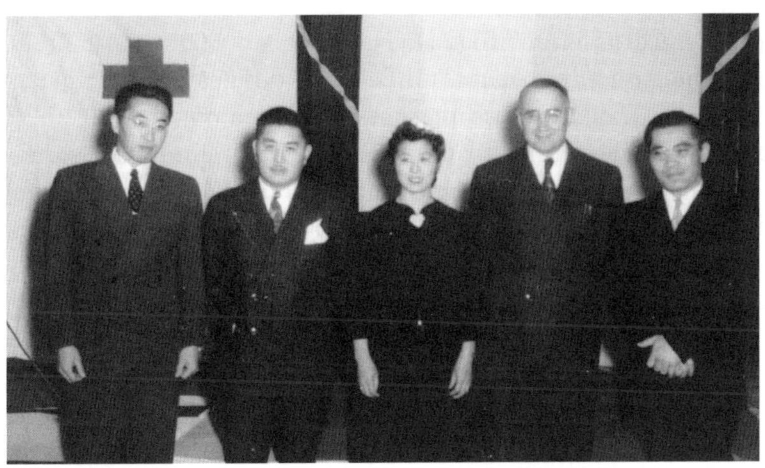

Topaz hospital party, December 29, 1944. Left to right: Drs. Henry Sugiyama, James Goto, Masako (Kusayanagi) Miura, Chief Medical Officer, probably Douglas R. Collier, MD, and Mr. Taira, a dental tech who the doctors taught to give anesthesia.

down to Manzanar.... He didn't like the fact that we didn't follow his orders and the patients listened to the doctors and not his instructions. The nurses also followed the Dr. Togasaki sisters and also paid no attention to his authority."

After being transferred to Manzanar, Yoshiye and Kazue would meet regularly with the assistant director, Kazue's former classmate. "As she saw us often, she would tell us that the camp situation was such that she could not see that things would improve. Administration was going to be a continuation of the current situation, so she advised us to leave as soon as we could make any satisfactory arrangements. At that time, Kazue and I decided that as long as we wouldn't be that effective in camp, we might be as well just get out. We probably could be more helpful outside."

Kazue went to Chicago to a Catholic hospital and received extra training in obstetrics for her residency. Yoshiye, on the other hand, headed for New York to Bellevue Hospital, where she had to repeat her internship and residency, despite her six years of training at Los Angeles County General Hospital before the war.

MASAMICHI "MAC" SUZUKI

Months later on July 15, 1943, Tule Lake was designated a segregation camp for "disloyals"—those internees who had answered "no, no" to the WRA's so-called loyalty questions. With 12,000 individuals transferred to Tule Lake from other camps and only 6,500 moving out, Tule Lake, overcrowded with close to 18,700 prisoners, was ripe for tension and dissension.

During the first week of November 1943, a series of events culminated in the takeover of the camp by the U.S. military. WRA director Dillon Myer had arrived on November 1 to investigate a general work strike of camp farm workers. Three hundred acres of vegetables were ready to be harvested, so the WRA recruited strikebreakers from the various camps, reportedly paying them one dollar an hour, compared to the $16 a month that the Tule Lake internees had been paid before.

Outraged, the internees formed a Negotiation Committee, which met with both Myer and the Project Director Raymond R. Best to air grievances. According to a 1943 WRA report prepared by John Bigelow, reports officer of the Minidoka Relocation Center, Negotiation Committee spokesman George Kuratomi made specific charges regarding the Tule Lake Hospital:

> a. Deplorable conditions at the hospital have caused the ire of the center residents.
> b. Dr. Pedicord made two appendicitis patients wait until it was almost too late.
> c. A person suffering from meningitis was refused care by a Caucasian doctor.
> d. A pregnant woman was given morphine injections which resulted in a still-birth.
> e. It has been said that some of the Caucasians [sic] doctors don't have licenses to practice medicine.
> f. Dr. Pedicord allows only one ambulance on Sunday for 18,000 people.
> g. Caucasian doctors neglected a two-year-old boy who had been scalded and as a result he died.

While WRA director Myer was talking over these and other related issues, Dr. Pedicord was attacked by some young internees in his private office at Tule Lake Hospital. According to a report prepared by John Bigelow, Pedicord was placed in a strangle hold, kicked, and beaten into semi-consciousness. His eyeglasses were "snatched" from his face and carefully put on a nearby shelf before the physical attack ensued.

The incident had occurred in the early afternoon, unbeknownst to Mac Suzuki. "I was playing bridge with some dentist friends over at their barrack," he recalled. "It must've been about nine o'clock [at night] or so, and I was coming back to the hospital, when I noticed [makes a staccato sound]; it was gunfire. I said to myself, 'What's going on?' And as I got closer to the hospital area, I noticed that there was a line of soldiers with their helmets and the guns and bayonets.

"And then the soldier said, 'Who goes there?'

"'This is Dr. Suzuki.'

"'Well,' he said, 'we've got an order that no one is to cross here.'

"And I said, 'Well, I live in the hospital.'

"And he said, 'Well, it doesn't make any difference.'

"And I asked, 'Would you call your officers, whoever is in command?'

"And so, I think there was a captain who came over, one of them, maybe it might have been a lieutenant, that came over.

"I explained the situation, and he said, 'All right, Doctor. You can [go].'

"So, I slipped back into the hospital. That night, nobody slept."

As Suzuki made his way through the hospital, he was able to witness the aftermath of the beating of Dr. Pedicord earlier that day. According to Suzuki, several apprehended Kibei suspects were lined up along a wall of one of the hospital wings. Their arms raised, they were being questioned by WRA authorities. Dr. Pedicord, meanwhile, had been taken out of camp to recuperate at a hotel in nearby Klamath Falls.

Dr. Pedicord returned to camp a few days later. "He was bruised. I think he had an arm in a sling, and I think his face was sort of black and blue, swollen. We were just amazed that he came back," said Suzuki.

He then issued his first order since December 1: "Line up the staff outside the hospital."

"And then, he started pointing out, 'You, you, you, I don't want you here in my hospital!'"

According to Suzuki, he pointed to practically every single doctor and medical student, including himself. For the next two days, Suzuki remained in his barracks. The situation seemed tenuous. The inmates were polarized into different political camps. Suzuki feared that if he went to the mess hall that he may be beaten or abused. As a result, he decided to forego meals. A couple of days later, there was a knock on the door of Suzuki's barracks. Suzuki was prepared: he had his baseball bat for protection.

"I asked, 'Who's at the door?'

"And he said, 'This is Captain So-and-so.'

"And I asked, 'What do you want?'

"He said, 'Well, I've got an order to take you out.'

"I said, 'Fine. Just give me five minutes to get dressed.'

"Once I got dressed, I got into a jeep with the captain and came out. And the following day after that, we got onto the train, and they took us out."

Most of the other Japanese American doctors also left. Dentists and other individuals difficult to replace stayed on. Some, including Dr. George Hashiba, apparently decided to remain in Tule Lake.

According to Sacramento resident Eucaly Shirai, Dr. Hashiba stayed at Tule Lake until the very end. "He was not only a superb surgeon but an activist who fought for better medical conditions for his internee patients. He had a large practice in Fresno before the war and returned to it when the camp closed. I remember as a child, my parents talking about people in Sacramento traveling to Fresno to have Dr. Hashiba perform their surgery."

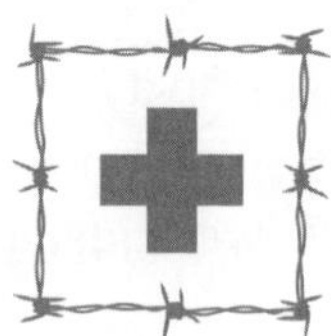

10. VISITORS FROM THE OUTSIDE

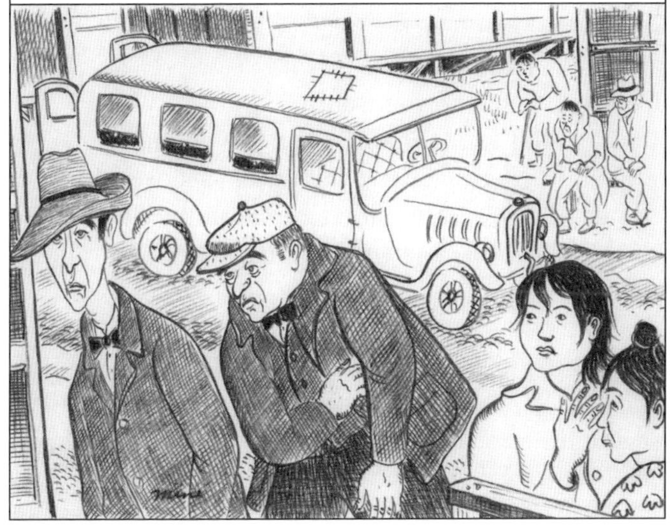

They stopped me and said, 'Oh, you owe us twenty-one dollars.'

—Sanbo Sakaguchi, MD, on leaving Manzanar after visiting his family

SANBO SAKAGUCHI

Dr. Sanbo Sakaguchi had not spent a day in camp until July 1944. Up to that summer, Sakaguchi, one of the seven Sakaguchi children raised on a farm in North Hollywood, had attended and graduated from Marquette School of Medicine in Milwaukee. He had also entered and completed a nine-month internship at Milwaukee County Hospital. Finally the government said that Sakaguchi would be allowed to visit his family in Manzanar in the summer of 1944.

He first stopped in Utah, where his father had been hospitalized for cancer of the nasal pharynx. "After treatment for a year, everything subsided, but then it came back. It started growing down the throat. He had to have a tracheotomy done, and he was in bad shape." From Utah, Sakaguchi took a train to Reno, Nevada, and traveled by bus on a back road to the concentration camp.

Apparently the camp administrators knew about Sakaguchi's upcoming visit and had plans for him. Dr. Teiji Takahashi, who had been operating the ear, nose, and throat (ENT) clinic, had been taken to Los Angeles County Hospital for surgery for colon cancer, which meant there was no ENT doctor for the entire camp.

"So when I got there, they said, 'Please help us out, help us out. Run the ear, nose and throat clinic.'

"So I spent about four or five hours a day running the ear, nose, and throat clinic.... The hospital was a small hospital; they were not that [well] equipped. If something real big came up, they had to send them out to either Los Angeles County or like my dad, they sent him to Salt Lake City, University of Utah Hospital. They didn't have any equipment for radiation treatment.... I just finished my internship, so I was a young doctor.... I felt I could do the work, but I wasn't that experienced."

For two weeks, Sakaguchi worked with the four other doctors on staff. On two Wednesdays, he and Dr. Morris Little, the hospital administrator, did ten tonsillectomies. During one of his examinations, he diagnosed a girl with acute appendicitis and together with a surgeon, operated on her.

"After being there two weeks, as I was leaving, I got to the gate where you get out.

"They stopped me and said, 'Oh, you owe us $21."

"I said, 'What for?'

"Your room and board... for the two weeks."

Sakaguchi considered calling the medical director and getting the fee waived, but the bus was on its way. There was no time for phone calls. So he paid the sentries the $21 rather than stay another day.

He left his family in Manzanar, unaware of a chain of tragic events that would strike his family members, one by one. "My oldest sister Chico had allergies, and she was allergic to dust. So when she got into camp, that made her allergies worse, and it turned into asthma. She got out of camp and was relocating to Philadelphia. While she was going to Philadelphia [she] had to stop in Chicago and be put in a hospital because she had a severe asthmatic attack." She eventually made it to Philadelphia, where she worked as a nursery school teacher, but succumbed to an overdose of adrenaline given for another asthmatic attack and died.

Within months, his father passed away in Manzanar. Then one of his older brothers, Obo, became ill. "My brother was one of the dentists in camp, [and] had developed stomach trouble. The radiologist, who wasn't a certified radiologist, fluoroscoped him and said there was nothing wrong. But actually, he was developing cancer of the stomach....

"So the day he was leaving camp, he was going to Philadelphia [to] relocate [there], and I think a day or two before he had a stomach ache. So they had to cancel the trip. They eventually sent him to Los Angeles County, because he developed a bowel obstruction. They sent him to county, and he was obstructed, really blown up....

"He finally went into shock, and they operated on him and found that he had cancer of the stomach that had metastasized through the intestines all over and down into the rectum. It also obstructed the ileo-cecum valve, the junction of the small and large bowel. So [in spite of] the surgery, he was just in too bad of shape, and he just didn't make it."

For one month, Sakaguchi traveled ten thousand miles from Milwaukee to Philadelphia to Los Angeles to Manzanar, to pick up the ashes of his deceased sister and to attend family funerals. "Being a doctor now and looking back, my dad must have had a tumor, a small tumor in the back of his throat. And because of all the dust in camp, I think that stimulated that tumor to grow."

JAMES YAMAZAKI

While James Yamazaki was completing his last year of medical school at Marquette, his parents had been moved approximately 1,775 miles from Santa Anita Assembly Center to the concentration camp in Jerome, Arkansas. On a few occasions, Yamazaki received anonymous phone calls while in Milwaukee: "Tell your dad to slow down, or he's going to be buried."

Yamazaki wasn't surprised that his father would engender such animosity. "[My dad] was convinced that having come here to the United States, that we were here to stay, that this was our home. So that in all the pictures of the church, there's always the church banner and the American flag. Even at picnics, in the old days."

In camp, where politics polarized the imprisoned Nikkei, Rev. Yamazaki took a strong position in supporting the conscription of Japanese American men. According to his son, he would tell young internees: "Well, after the war, if you want to have a place here, this would be your only way—to do the same thing as the Jones' boys on the street were doing. Then you might be more acceptable when the war is over."

Indeed, the minister's detractors followed up on their threats. Rev. Yamazaki was beaten in Jerome on early March 1943. James Yamazaki had no idea of what had transpired until he visited the camp after his graduation from medical school. Arriving in the darkness of night "in the middle of nowhere," Yamazaki was met by a military detachment who took him to his father, who was recuperating in the hospital.

"He was all bandaged up... he said, 'How are you?' He started joking and said, 'Hey, look at my toe, I can move them.'

"So he was joking like that. He always had a thing about his toes. You know, Jesus washing the feet and all that."

With his father in the Jerome hospital, Yamazaki stayed with his mother in their barracks. He remained in Jerome for about ten days and was asked by the medical staff to give a talk on snakes and herpetology, a field that Yamazaki had studied during college, since the discovery of snakes in the former swampland was common.

For their safety, his father and mother were eventually moved to Chicago, where Rev. Yamazaki became active in assisting Japanese Americans resettle after they left camp. When asked whether his father knew who his assailants were, Yamazaki replied, "He knew who they were, but he never told me. All I know is ... when they came back to California, the [St. Mary's] rectory was sort of a hostel. All kinds of people were staying in every room because they had nowhere to go. Some of the [people] that beat him came to the rectory and stayed here. But he wouldn't tell me who they were."

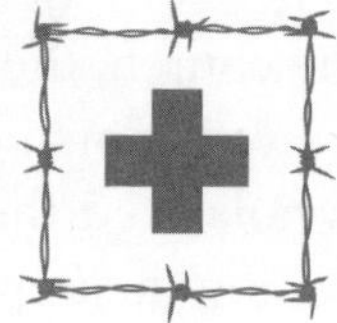

11. EARLY EXITS TO THE OUTSIDE

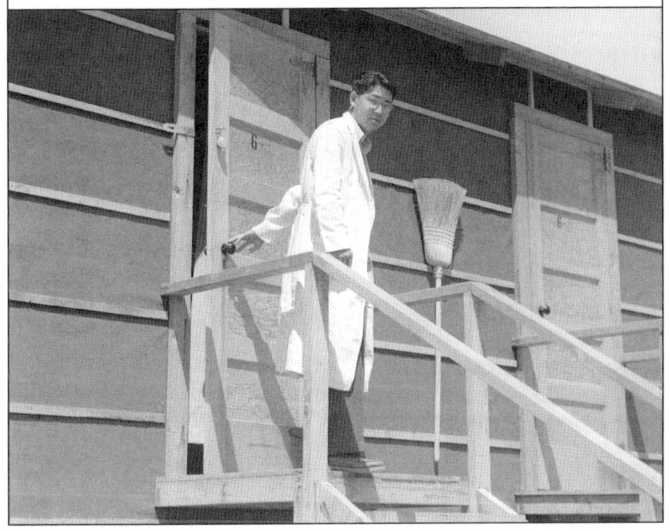

I didn't know even if they'd let us go out, until my brother went out. Then I picked it up, and decided I was going to have to hurry and get out too.

—William Sato, MD, who was incarcerated with his family in Gila River War Relocation Center in Arizona

For the first three weeks in March 1942, Japanese Americans on the West Coast could move into the nation's interior–provided that they could identity identify non-Japanese sponsors. Facing severe racial hostility and limited financial resources, only a few families found this a viable option. Once incarcerated, some inmates were able to get permission from the WRA to leave camp as early as the end of 1942. Closely investigated and cleared, these individuals moved east to work or attend school. The Quaker-supported American Friends Service Committee established the National Japanese American Student Relocation Council to help young Nisei leave camp to pursue their college degrees. Some Nisei felt that they needed to stay behind in camp to assist their non-English-speaking parents.

WILLIAM SATO

William Sato, in his early twenties, watched his younger siblings leave Gila River War Relocation Center, one by one. His brother George left in December 1942 for his premed program at Washington University, followed by their sister Jane, who attended Rochester University to train as a nurse.

Sato, on the other hand, said, "[I] lost my direction to go into medicine. I thought maybe I'd never be able to do that.... Being in camp you know, and not [knowing] what the future's going to be like. You don't know what they're going to do to us, for one."

When asked whether he was depressed at the time, William answered, "Oh sure, sure I was. Although not to the point where I couldn't do anything. You know I went out and looked for a job and things like that. Depression, yes...I didn't fight to get out of camp as much as my brother did....I didn't know even if they'd let us go out, until my brother went out. Then I picked it up, and decided I was going to have to hurry and get out too."

Through some help offered by the Quaker organization, the American Friends Service Committee, Sato applied to three medical schools and was quickly accepted into Loyola University in Chicago. In the winter of 1943, Sato and his wife, with WRA, FBI, and other releases in hand, were driven out of Gila to the train station at Coolidge, a small Arizona railroad station. But there they experienced more hurdles:

"The trainmaster there wouldn't sell us a ticket...I said, 'Here's the money. Here's the release. I [have] a permit to leave camp. Give me my ticket.'

"I handed him the money. He wouldn't take the money. I turned to the escort that brought us there, and I said, 'Hey, intervene or something.'

"All he [said] was, 'It's not my business.'...

"So I turned to my wife, and said, 'It looks like we're going back into camp.'

"Here you could hear the train coming down. They made a stop at that station, either took on something or left something. It was just about ready to start up again when this trainmaster gave us the tickets....

"I guess he was going to teach us a lesson or something like that. So that's the send-off from camp we had."

SAKAYE SHIGEKAWA

While Dr. Shigekawa was in Santa Anita Assembly Center, she wrote several letters to the government that she wanted to be released. Finally before the temporary detention center closed in October, a public health official was dispatched to Santa Anita. During the official's visit, Shigekawa repeated that she wanted to leave. When she was told that she would be moved to Heart Mountain Relocation Center, she flatly refused to work and explained that she had a colleague, Dr. Ann Patras, who was willing to house her in Chicago. For whatever reason, the authorities agreed to let Shigekawa go.

Upon her arrival to Chicago, she applied for a residency at Walter Memorial Hospital and was accepted with an offer of $150 a month. However, the hospital ended up paying her much less. "I was kind of resentful for that because they promised me," said Shigekawa. "So there was another doctor, a woman doctor, that used to come to the hospital, and she asked me if I would like to work with her.

"At first I felt obliged to the hospital for taking me at the time they did. Then I thought, 'No, why should I?' So I didn't even let them know that I was leaving.

"[As] I was walking [out], the superintendent of the hospital said, 'Where are you going?'

"I said, 'I'm leaving.'

"So then he said, 'Well, you know, we took you in place of a man.'

"Under my breath I thought, 'Well, there aren't any men around.'

"That didn't work, so then he said, 'Well, you know there's a war on.'

"I said, 'Yes, and I didn't start it,' and I walked away."

HOMER YASUI

Homer Yasui had spent a total of only four months in detention camps–first at Pinedale Assembly Center and then Tule Lake Relocation Center–when he considered going to college in the nation's interior.

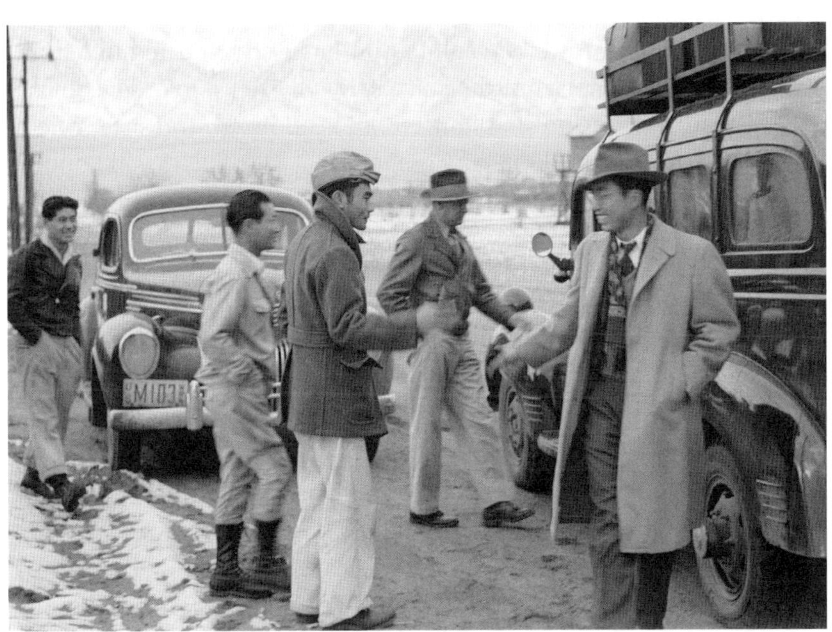

Departing the Manzanar Relocation Center

Although he and his other Nisei classmates from Hood River High School's Class of 1942 had missed their graduation ceremonies, principal Herman Kramer had mailed diplomas to all fourteen of them in Tule Lake. "So we missed the last month of school. But Mr. Kramer said, 'Well, it's not their fault that they couldn't attend school,'" said Yasui.

Equipped with his high school diploma, Yasui began the process of applying to four-year colleges. According to Yasui family biographer Lauren Kessler, this idea was suggested and heartily endorsed by his mother Shidzuyo, "who was becoming increasingly alarmed by Homer's behavior."

"One of the things I did there that summer was play a ton of baseball. Baseball was a big thing and camp dances were another big thing at Tule Lake. So it wasn't all work for me by any means. Because remember, I was a seventeen-year-old thoughtless, non-thinking young boy, having a great time in camp. I think I kind of made my mother despair about where I was headed for, because she's the one, I'm sure, that got me out of camp to go to college."

Outside of camp were Yasui's ambitious and educated older siblings. Attorney Minoru had defied curfew and exclusion orders during World War II, while brother Shu, whom he idolized, and sister Michi were studying at the University of Denver. As a result, Yasui applied and was accepted to the same university, but only if some requirements were fulfilled:

"[The universities] had to have assurances that my parents had enough money to pay for the tuition, and had to have a guarantee of lodging, had to have clearance from the security quarters like the FBI and the armed forces. So there's a lot of hoops to jump through, but I don't remember doing it. So I think, 'Well golly, my brother must have done that,' [Roku], the one that's nearly ten years older than me."

Taking a bus from Tule Lake with three other Nisei, Yasui traveled to Denver. He "felt kind of bad leaving because theoretically I was the man of the family. Although when I look back on the record, I was not listed as the head of the family. My mother was."

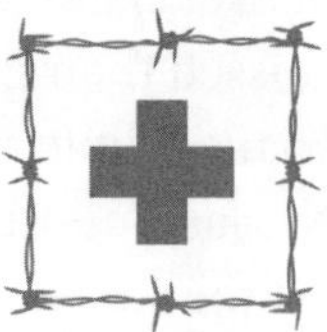

12. “I AM PROUD TO SERVE”

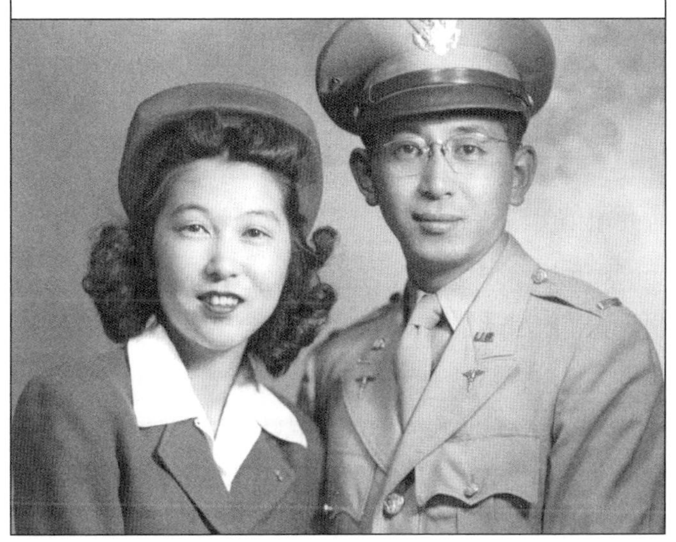

. . . in a few hours we had collected about twenty-eight truckloads full of kids.

—James Yamazaki, MD, who was a medic with the 106th Infantry Division during the Battle of the Bulge, the last major German offensive on the Western Front

The most well-known all-Nisei military units during World War II were the 100th Infantry Battalion, comprised of mostly young men in Hawaii, and the 442d Regimental Combat Team, another all-Nisei unit which included soldiers who either volunteered or were drafted from detention. Some Nisei had been drafted prior to the bombing of Pearl Harbor, and their status was often in limbo as they were classified for some time as 4-C, or enemy alien. One exception was Dr. James Yamazaki, a medic who was the only Asian American in the 106th Infantry Division.

ROBERT S. KINOSHITA
AUGUSTUS "GUS" TANAKA

A Hawai'i-born physician experienced in working for the military, Dr. Robert Kinoshita was an inspiration to eighteen-year-old Augustus "Gus" Tanaka, who had just entered Reed College in Portland when the war broke out. Although his own father was a doctor, Tanaka decided to pursue medicine because of his association with Kinoshita at the Portland Assembly Center.

"While I was at the camp, Dr. Kinoshita was my mentor and showed [me] the ropes of simple things. He and a couple of the nurses taught me how to make beds and how to bathe patients. I think they allowed me to do a lot of things that orderlies in a normal situation wouldn't be allowed to do, because of the primitive situation and the shortage of help there. But Dr. Robert Kinoshita is the one I think, and Dr. [Robert] Shiomi also did a lot to kind of inspire my interest in medicine."

After Kinoshita and his family were moved to the Wyoming Heart Mountain Relocation Center, a 150-bed hospital, encompassing seventeen barracks, was eventually opened. The hospital serviced 130 outpatients a day; by the end of the war, 1,000 operations and 566 births would have taken place. In addition to his medical duties, Kinoshita had been active in establishing the only officially recognized USO Club of all the camps in Heart Mountain's Block 23. Meanwhile, the army captain continued to volunteer for active military duty.

For a period of time, Japanese Americans, all US citizens, were classified 4-C, or enemy alien. They were barred from being sent overseas to fight on behalf of the United States. "He was also trying to serve in any manner that he thought possible," explained his son Richard. "He wrote letters to the local and international Red Cross, volunteering to work for free, and was turned down. He wrote a letter to the governor of Wyoming, Governor Hunt, asking to be placed on a selective service board as he had been in Oregon. The governor sent that request to the Wyoming medical examiner's office, who simply said that they didn't think anybody would want to work with a Japanese, whether he was qualified as a doctor or a citizen of the United States. But the governor's letter to my father was worded much nicer than that, much more polite. So that was turned down.

"Upon learning that the United States government was going to activate a Nisei fighting outfit, Dad volunteered. He was among the first fifteen hundred volunteers from the camps to be accepted. He took his physical at Fort Warren, Cheyenne, Wyoming, and passed. He was reactivated as a captain in the United States Army." Before he left Heart Mountain, he gave a speech, "I Am Proud to Serve," which was published in the *Heart Mountain Sentinel* on March 6, 1943:

> My commission as an officer of the United States Army bears a phrase which says the President "reposing special trust and confidence in the patriotism, valor, fidelity and abilities" of the applicant appoints him to the position. I am gratified that I have been given an opportunity to actively carry out that trust placed upon me at a time when my nation is in danger.
>
> We evacuees have been through a great deal in the past year. We have shared the pain of evacuation and the trials of readjustment in this strange place. Now we are given the chance to prove the loyalty that we have declared so often. It is a challenge to our faith and patriotism.
>
> Some of you may be embittered by your experiences, but I do not feel that way. Since the declaration of war I have offered my services innumerable times, even as a buck private, and I feel that my efforts are now at last rewarded.
>
> I consider this my opportunity to prove that I am worthy of my American heritage. I am proud to serve my country, and I would be ashamed of myself, and my people, if we could not meet this challenge.
>
> I want my children to be proud of me as a soldier of my country, and when the war is over, I will want to be able to stand before any man and tell him that I too helped to bring victory to America. I have faith in the future of the United States.
>
> I am proud that I will be associated with hundreds and thousands of other nisei in this great crusade for the freedom and liberty of the common man, and I invite others who have not made up their minds to join us in our battle. This great nation has given us life. It is the least we can do in her time of need to offer ourselves in her service.

The Kinoshita family left for Camp McCoy, Wisconsin, where the 100th Battalion, made up of mostly Hawaiian Nisei, were training. Then the operation was moved to Camp Shelby, Mississippi–training grounds for the all-Nisei 442nd Regimental Combat Team (RCT). "When my father was accepted for duty...all of these men had to go through special investigations. He had been told that he would become the executive medical officer for the 442nd, which would be the second-in-command. When he arrived, he found out that, like the black units in the United States Army, there were going to be white officers appointed over any other officer. Instead of becoming the executive medical officer, they gave him the title of medical planning and training officer."

For one year, Captain Kinoshita trained the medics of the 442nd. "Strangely, part of his duties included keeping the two sides, the Hawaiian boys and the stateside Nisei, separated sometimes, because when they first got together there was such a culture clash," explained Richard. "The Hawaiian boys were so outgoing, and they thought that the mainland Nisei were stuffy and trying to lord it over them because they were educated. That was not the case. Dad was able to bridge that because he was born and raised in Hawaii but educated in the United States.

"There were problems. Mississippi was a segregationist state. There immediately rose some problems because, quite frankly, the Mississippi officials did not know how to treat Orientals. So it was decided that for the duration of the 442nd's stay at Shelby that the Oriental troops would be considered white, and my father had to, all the officers had to, tell their men that for the duration they would be considered white. My father remembered that some of them actually cheered because they thought they were getting a break. But when they thought about it, [they] realized that this was just for the short period they were going to be there."

As it turned out, the 442nd had too many doctors and dentists as so many Nisei medical professionals had either volunteered or been drafted for military service. Dr. Shigeru Hara was assigned to the Sixth Army and served in stateside medical facilities, overseeing eight wards at one time. He also was sent to France where he worked with soldiers with malaria. Another young Nisei, Iwao George Kawakami, was immediately drafted upon his graduation from undergraduate premed studies at Washington University in St. Louis in mid-1944. Putting his medical education at Rochester University on hold, he entered basic training in Texas and was eventually shipped to Italy to be part of the Occupation of Europe. Italy and Yugoslavia were still in conflict, and he became a medic and joined a tank battalion. He was eventually transferred to the 442nd Regimental Combat Team. Later through his military service, Kawakami had his medical education financed by the GI bill.

In summer 1944, Gus Tanaka would also have his own military experience. Upon his status being reclassified from 4-C to 1-A (able-bodied male), he was drafted within a week. He first trained at Camp Blanding, Texas, to serve as a replacement for the 442nd Regimental Combat Team, but was eventually sent to the University of Minnesota to enroll in the Army Specialized Training Program (ASTP) to prepare soldiers for the Occupation of Japan. The University of Minnesota, ironically, had previously declined to accept Tanaka because of the university's military contracts.

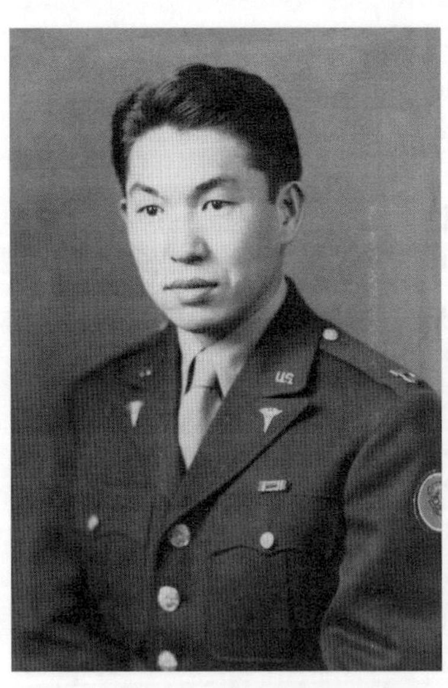

JAMES YAMAZAKI

Dr. James Yamazaki was called to active duty in 1944, after he had completed an internship at St. Louis City Hospital in Missouri. Before he reported to the U.S. Army Medical Field Service School at Carlisle Barracks in Pennsylvania, he stopped by New York to court and marry a young Nisei woman, Aki Hirashiki. Before they could enjoy newlywed life, Yamazaki left with the 106th "Roaring Lions" Infantry Division for England and Germany.

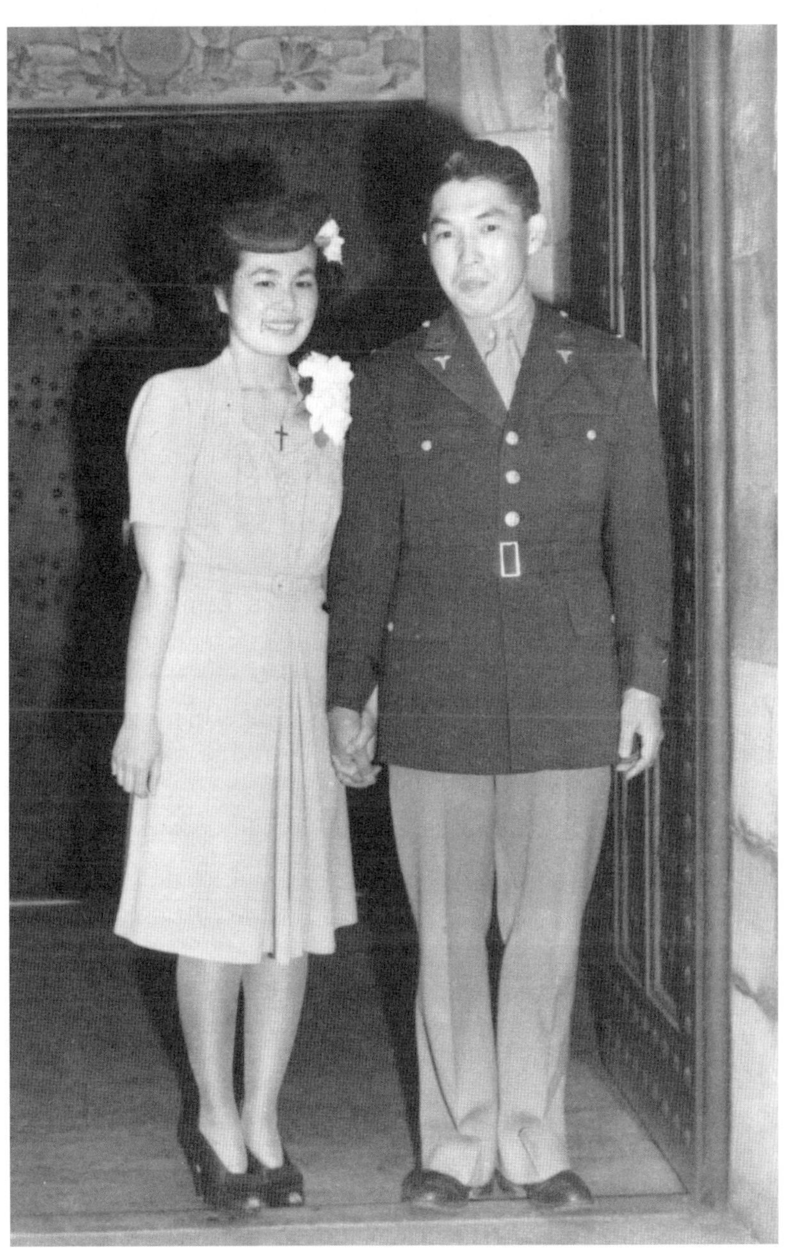

Dr. and Mrs. James N. Yamazaki at their wedding,
Grace Episcopal Church, New York City, April 1, 1944.

The only Asian American in the 106th Division, the twenty-seven-year-old Yamazaki found himself amidst teenage infantry soldiers. It was his responsibility as battalion surgeon to accompany these young men to the front lines of combat. Since D-Day had passed, the unit thought they were going to be sent to a "quiet sector." Experienced infantry soldiers had been shipped out, and their replacements turned out to be those training to be officers.

"So we were always examining the officers," said Yamazaki. "They would come in and say, 'Hey, I've really got a bad back...and I'm not fit for service.'

"So I'd write down, 'Not fit for service.' I didn't want them next to me fighting.

"The general said, 'You can't do that. We need them.'

"'Even the guys with the stiff arms?' I said.

"'Yes. Take them all.'

"'One eye?'

"'Yes. That's okay. One eye is good. Just take them all.'"

Within five days, the "quiet sector" quickly transformed itself into the bloodiest last major battle on the Western Front, which later came to be known as the Battle of the Bulge. In mid-December 1944, the German army—five hundred thousand soldiers—made a last ditch effort and tried to push through the Ardennes region of Belgium and Luxembourg. The 106th medic team had only a three-quarter quarter-ton truck and a Jeep. "This was just a first aid kind of thing. When you have hundreds of guys knocked out, you have nothing left. So all you could do is just collect them and do whatever you can." Medical supplies were quickly depleting. The enemy was overwhelming the American troops. "A division consists of twelve thousand men, and we had other supporting units. And you put a certain amount, about a fifth of them in reserve, so there were about ten thousand men on the line. Out of that ten thousand, seven thousand were casualties within five days." The first aid station was set up on a mountainside. Whenever someone asked for a medic, the aid men were dispatched to even the heaviest combat areas. Trapped in the Ardennes forest, the eight thousand of the 106th unit were either captured or killed. Yamazaki's life was spared, but he was taken as a prisoner of war (POW). Before they left the battlefield, he and other American GIs loaded German trucks with the wounded. "In a few hours we had collected about twenty-eight truckloads full of kids," said Yamazaki.

"But then the Germans said after a few hours, 'That's it.' So we left a lot of them in the snow."

From there, Yamazaki and the other prisoners walked fifteen miles to a German town called Koblenz. Loaded into boxcars, they were taken by train to a POW camp in Hanover. On their way there the POW trains encountered fire from the Allied Forces. "As we approached, we could hear the planes getting louder and louder. This would be about three or four days after we were captured. Then the bombs started to drop.... And the [German] guys locked us into the boxcars. We could see them running toward the shelters.... it's impossible to let us out. You can hear the sirens. They had a cadence. As the planes get closer, the intervals of blasts get closer and closer, and finally it's one continuous sound of the sirens. That's when the bombs are really falling, and the boxcars are jumping up and down.... When we got the all-clear, we were still there. But we don't know what happened to the other guys–the guys in our outfit that we left together for Koblenz. I never met up. When we got to the first POW camp, there was nobody from my outfit. I was the only one."

Yamazaki was moved from one POW camp to another. With the Germans themselves suffering from depleted supplies, the prisoners were fed only rotten potatoes. Imprisoned for a total of five months, he lost fifty pounds.

"It was about Christmas time, and the Germans said, 'Hey, we're going to bring something. Christmas goodies.' And they kept [saying] this... And we thought, 'What rot.'

"But sure enough one day, they came with boxes filled with stuff including wine." In the next compound, separated by only barbed wire, were Russian prisoners. One segment of the American POWs thought, "Hey, we're supposed to be buddies with them, let's share it."

The other side said, "Hey, we may not have another bite of food to eat again."

"'It's us or them, right?'

"So we said, 'Let's have a vote. We're going to share or not share.'

"It was, 'no.'"

Shortly thereafter came St. Nicholas Day, the Russian holiday. "The Germans let it be known that they're going to bring food to the Russians," said Yamazaki. "So we said, 'Maybe they don't like the Russians; there are bad feelings.' But they did bring it to them. The next day, the Russians, all spit and polished as best they could under those conditions, came in and shared their gifts with us!"

During his captivity, Yamazaki bathed only two or three times. "We went through the delousing showers, but by then we heard about the Holocaust, and when we went through the chambers, we didn't know what was going to happen.... Yes, so it was good to see these guys coming out of the [showers] because we were near Dachau."

Meanwhile, Aki was left alone in New York to wonder where her husband was. "But she did know I was okay because when I was in this first POW camp, they said, 'We're going to have one of you guys broadcast back to the States. We'll take you to the broadcast booth.' And they said, 'So you write your message.'" The soldiers did, even though they thought it was just a ploy. "But they did read my message over the wire. [My wife Aki] got letters from people who heard it over the short wave." Up to that point, Aki, who was staying in New York, had no idea what had happened to her husband. Because of the 106th's debilitating losses, nothing had been heard from a member of the battalion up to that time. "I counted about twenty notes saying they heard that Jim was okay," said Aki.

After one failed rescue attempt, Yamazaki was finally liberated and eventually returned to the U.S. in June 1945. He then obtained pediatric residencies with children's hospitals in Pennsylvania and Cincinnati. He was honorably discharged from the army as a captain in March 1946. But his connection to World War II and its aftermath did not end there. He was recruited to serve as a pediatrician with the Atomic Bomb Casualty Commission (ABCC) to investigate the long-term effects of the atomic bombs. Also joining ABCC on a different research project was Dr. Mac Suzuki.

KATSUMI JAMES NAKADATE

In 1942, Dr. Katsumi James Nakadate left Eloise Hospital in Michigan for East Chicago. Once there, he sent for his fiancée, Mary Marumoto, a former Portland Rose Festival Queen, who was interned in Minidoka Relocation Center in Idaho. They were married in a small parsonage in Indiana and honeymooned at the Military Intelligence Service Language School in Minnesota, where Mary's brother was undergoing training. Within five months, Captain Nakadate would receive his orders to report to Pennsylvania for medical army training. An assignment to Camp Shelby, Mississippi, the training camp for the 442d Regimental Combat Team, soon followed. At Shelby, Nakadate would meet Dr. Robert Kinoshita. Approximately five medics were assigned to the regiment but with the shortage of doctors, Nakadate was transferred to the Sixty-ninth Division as a Battalion Aid Station doctor and one month later, to the Seventeenth Airborne, a parachute unit. "...I was the only American of Japanese descent in the whole division, I think, and then of course, with the battalion, I was the only battalion doctor. They took care of me real well; they didn't know when they might need me. They took care of me one-hundred percent."

Ordered to the front where the Battle of the Bulge was raging, the Seventeenth Airborne were flown from England to France. Then the battalion entered the front line on jeeps. "I had a jeep, two jeeps, and a trailer on the back end. That was our group, where we were moving, once we were out of the air. I had my medical supplies in the trailer behind one of the jeeps, and I sat in the other jeep on the front seat next to the driver with some medical supplies in the back seat."

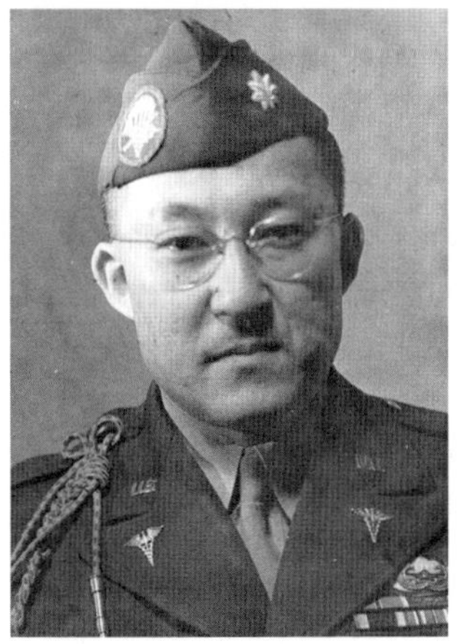

"We moved so fast, we didn't go to any mess hall or anything like that. We had to eat in the jeep; I had to eat while we were moving...those little packages, K rations," said Nakadate, who explained that he broke a tooth during one of their bumpy rides.

"The thing that bothered me most was when I was traveling in the jeep, because I had to work maybe all day and part of the night in the aid station, when I was in the jeep, I'd fall asleep. My driver, who was a wonder[ful] fellow—they gave him sergeant's stripes, three chevrons—he was my driver. He'd grab me so that I wouldn't fall out of the jeep while I was sleeping. Finally he tied a rope across the jeep so he wouldn't have to grab hold of me to keep me in the jeep. How many times he saved me, I don't know. But the only problem with that was, I couldn't jump out of the jeep if somebody started to shoot at me. The Germans would put a rope across the road, on trees to behead people in jeeps. Because our jeep was always open: all it was, was a windshield. Part of the time, they'd take the windshield down because it'd shine.... it could tell the German people that there was somebody coming."

Dr. Nakadate's first priority was to pick up the wounded on the front lines. "The only thing I could possibly do if they were bleeding was to maybe stop the bleeding. The worst thing was that I had to pick up somebody that was dead.... And if they weren't bad, why then I'd use my jeep to put the stretchers on and send them back to the nearest—not a hospital—but the nearest division medical team."

Dealing with the mortally wounded—both Allied and Axis soldiers–would take its toll on Nakadate. "I always think about how tough it was, because our fellows would say, 'God is with us,' when they were wounded especially.

"And I'd say, 'God with you.'

"Not only that but the Germans would leave their wounded as they fled, and they'd leave their wounded. And do you know what their wounded men would say, '*Gott mit uns*.'

"I said, 'Is that the same god that our boys talk about?'... My religion would hurt a little bit then. 'God is with us,' or [as] the Germans say, '*Gott mit uns*.' Is that the same god? And here they were trying to kill each other; I'm trying to save their lives, whether they were German or whether they were American boys."

Nakadate did the best he could for the injured German soldiers. "The only time that I had a problem was they'd leave an officer, a dead German officer... taped so that they would blow up or something.

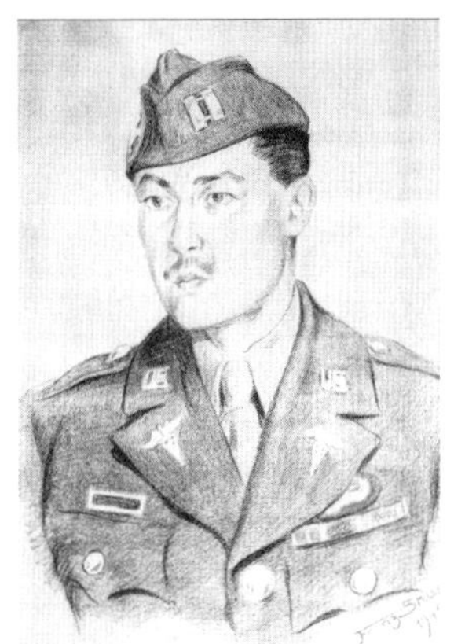

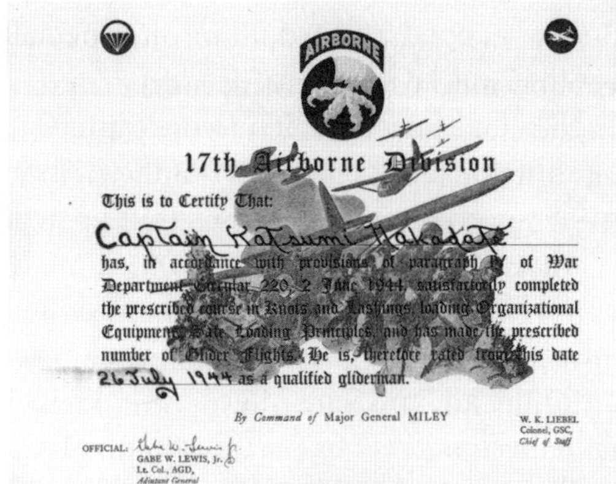

AIRBORNE

17th Airborne Division

This is to Certify That:

Captain Katsumi Nakadate

has, in accordance with provisions of paragraph [illegible] of War Department Circular 220, 2 June 1944, satisfactorily completed the prescribed course in Knots and Lashings, loading Organizational Equipment, Safe Loading Principles, and has made the prescribed number of Glider Flights. He is, therefore rated from this date 26 July 1944 as a qualified gliderman.

By Command of Major General MILEY

W. K. LIEBEL
Colonel, GSC,
Chief of Staff

OFFICIAL: GABE W. LEWIS, Jr.
Lt. Col., AGD,
Adjutant General

Clockwise from top left: Drawing of Dr. Katsumi J. Nakadate by a German soldier, Berlin, 1945; Capt. Nakadate's U.S Airborne Division qualification; Dr. Mary Oda and her husband, James; William Sato, MD, on his armored vehicle, prepared to forestall any violence during Italy's first democratic elections, Livorno, Italy, 1946.

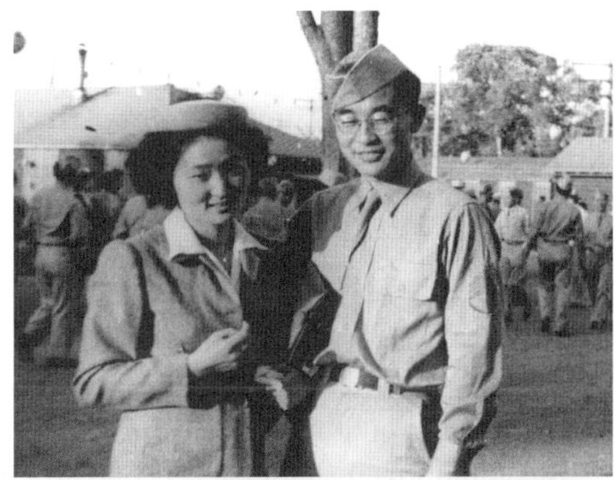

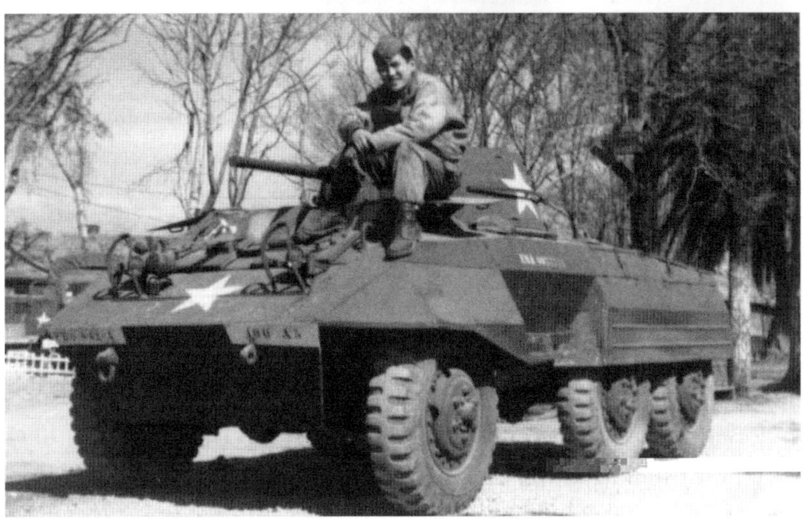

Booby-trapped, so I would never especially look for a German officer that was laying there."

Nakadate knew that if he were captured, that he would most likely be shot because he was part of the Airborne forces. He did, in fact, suffer several injuries from exploding artillery.

"*Bang!* And a piece of it would hit me. I got hit... right above my eye." Nakadate was also hit in front of his ear and in his neck. "But the worst injury I got was in my back when I was on a glider... I got hit in the air, and when I got out, I knew I was hurt and real bad. I didn't realize it, but by the time they had taken me, I must have fainted while I was taking care of people. The people didn't quite know it.

"I said, 'I hurt, I hurt, but you hurt worse than I...'

"And I took care of them until I must have fainted. Then the commanding officer of our group from where it was, said they were going to have to evacuate me, but we were across the river, the Rhine River. They had to take me back across the river when it was under control."

Shrapnel pinched his sciatic nerve. He could hardly walk, so he was placed on a stretcher and carried to the first aid station. "When they found that I was hurting back there, they had to take off my pants, and my pants were soaked with blood.... When they finally checked my blood later on, they said, 'You're anemic. You lost all that blood.'"

Nakadate was hospitalized in Belgium and later moved to facilities in France and England. He was in a British hospital during VE Day. Instead of returning to the United States, Nakadate opted to stay in Europe and was assigned to the occupation forces in Berlin. Finally at the end of 1945, Nakadate was sent back home on a tramp streamer. As it neared the East Coast of the United States, the Statue of Liberty in New York was visible to all the passengers.

"Well, I'm almost home," Nakadate said.

YOSHIYE TOGASAKI

After spending two years at Bellevue Hospital in New York, Dr. Yoshiye Togasaki was ready to move on. Despite the cold and even "belligerent" reception she faced from staff members, she gained much as a research assistant in pediatrics and from observing the work within a psychiatric unit for children. But now a new adventure was calling her: a new government program, the United Nations Relief and Rehabilitation Administration. Commissioned a captain in the army, Dr. Togasaki prepared for her mission to Europe to observe the aftermath of World War II.

"We were on the ocean for about four weeks. It was slow because we were zigzagging. I suddenly found that my professional services were needed because a young fellow had fallen out of bed and cut his lip up to his nose. By the time I saw him, he was bleeding profusely but we managed. I had never expected to do anything as delicate as sewing up the lip and nose together.

"With the use of sulfa drugs, we were most fortunate that we did not have any infection afterwards. When we docked in Italy, Naples, he was doing fine. Later I was on liberty attending one of the departmental meetings in Naples, and as I was walking the streets, someone stopped me. I didn't know why. He was in uniform—this was the person I had taken care of. He said, 'Doc, you don't know what you did for me. Look.' It was a perfect fit—you can hardly notice it. He only had a thin scar."

Togasaki finally arrived at a little town called Santa Maria Al Bagno, an old seaside resort in Puglia where the United Nations had established a small camp. "The refugees were being sent in very rapidly by the hundreds. It was our responsibility to take care of them. There was no food problem. The problem was the personal supplies like bed and mattress, blankets for individuals. Very often we would be short until we received them the next day."

Although supplies came regularly from Rome, tempers were short. After surviving wartime atrocities, refugees expected to have all their needs met by the camp administrators.

"They would become angry and demonstrate when they didn't have something they thought they should have," observed Dr. Togasaki. "This was a reaction to their long imprisonment and severity of their treatment when they were imprisoned. Some came from death camps such as Auschwitz.... They had seen their own families destroyed, killed, or physically put alive in ovens. Behavior was unpredictable [but] the social workers were doing well."

After six months, Dr. Togasaki was moved from Santa Maria to Lecce, the capital of the Italian province and headquarters for the southern camps which extended from Bari down to Santa Maria di Léuca. Conditions were good, and it was Dr. Togasaki's responsibility to check in on all the hospitals in the area. "Our clinic was one of the best stocked because friends sent in different items that were requested by us. The ladies in Berkeley would send in complete layettes—one after the other—for babies that were born. It meant a great deal to the mothers."

Dr. Togasaki completed her tour of duty in 1946. She then returned to San Francisco, where she began work as an assistant health officer and medical field worker for the state's Crippled Children's Services program, which included maternal and child health service.

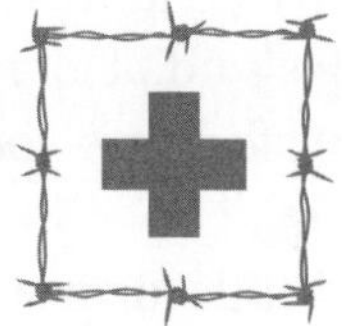

13. LAST DAYS OF CAMP

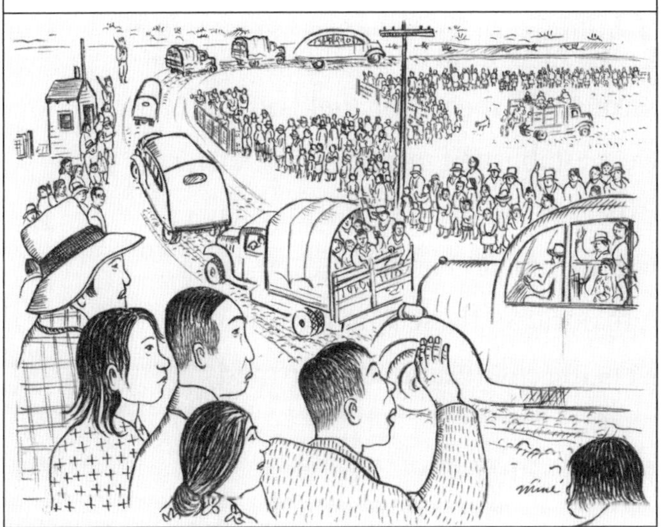

Here they're getting high wages, and we worked like slaves with nothing.

—Nurse Emi (Somekawa) Beckwith regarding the relationship of white and Japanese American nurses in Minidoka Relocation Center in Idaho

As the WRA was determined to scatter and assimilate Japanese Americans throughout the nation, field offices were established in cities like Denver, Chicago, and New York City. By 1944, 35,000 inmates had left the ten camps. A majority of those who remained were the elderly and the infirmed.

MASAKO (KUSAYANAGI) MIURA

Dr. Masako (Kusayanagi) Miura and her husband, Dr. James Goto, were among the few physicians who spent the entire duration of the war behind barbed wire. "Because when we were out there toward the end, all the Nisei doctors went into the army, and there wasn't anybody left to help out with the older Japanese," said Miura, who was incarcerated in Topaz until early September 1945. "So being short of doctors, the government sent in a lot of the German refugees, doctors from Germany. Of course, their English was with an accent, and it was hard to understand. They spoke no Japanese. So how would Issei be able to communicate with them?...

"So we figured we might as well stay and help out these people because otherwise they would really be in a pickle."

In Topaz, too, a shooting resulted in the death of an inmate—an old man with his dog. "I don't know if he was blind or what, but probably hard of hearing. Because when the MPs told him to halt, I guess he didn't hear him, and he kept walking around in the yard there. I guess he wasn't supposed to be in that yard. But he kept walking his dog around, and so the MP out there shot him. He keeled over and died."

GEORGE TARO AKAMATSU
HENRY IWAO SUGIYAMA

Doctors witnessed first-hand the turmoil during the transfer of people from other camps to Tule Lake Segregation Center. One was a native of Hiroshima, Japan, Dr. George Taro Akamatsu. Akamatsu had had been in his fourth year of family practice in Walnut Grove, a Japanese community near Sacramento, when the war broke out. Although he requested to be evacuated with the other Sacramento physicians, there were not enough doctors in the Seattle area, and the WCCA moved he and his wife Yasuka to Washington state, where Akamatsu assisted with medical examinations of internee families. They were then taken to Puyallup Assembly Center near Tacoma, Washington, before being moved to Tule Lake Relocation Center.

Yasuka Akamatsu described their experience at Tule Lake while

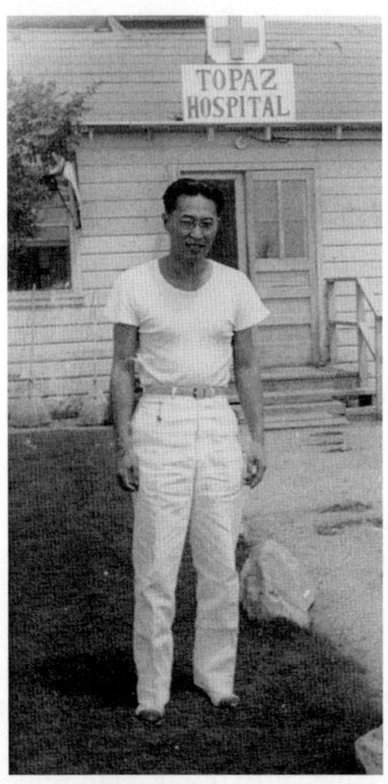

Dr. Henry Sugiyama in front of Topaz hospital.

it was in the process of changing to a more tightly controlled and patrolled segregation center: "The outgoing medical staff had to stay until [the transfer] was completed. The day we were told to get ready to move, no one came after us. Evidently, there were some commotions in the administration area, which caused the changes. We had to stay in our barracks for two more weeks. In the meantime, the administration was planning a way to get all of us scheduled to leave, out in one day."

Dr. Henry Sugiyama wasn't thinking of moving out of Tule Lake. "I wanted to stay in Tule because it was a bigger camp, and there were more variety of medical treatments, surgical treatments. Anyway, medicine would be a lot more interesting because we were crowded there. But they said, 'You can't stay here, because you're a 'yes-yes,' and if the 'no-nos' ever get a hold of you alone someplace, they're going to beat you to death.'

"So they had guards around my barrack.

"They said, 'Now you've got to leave.'"

From there, Sugiyama, his wife, and newborn moved to Topaz in Utah. "I did all the deliveries. I did the prenatal care. I did the postnatal care. I took care of the whole TB ward. I gave all the pneumothorax therapy to people that needed it.... I took care of the internal medicine, most of it anyway, and I helped in surgery. I was busy."

While Sugiyama was in Tule Lake, his mother was diagnosed with stomach cancer. His father was still incarcerated in Santa Fe alien detention camp. By the time the family moved to Topaz, "... [my mother] was dying. Then I had the chief medical officer of the camp, and we wrote to Washington, D.C., and said how about releasing him

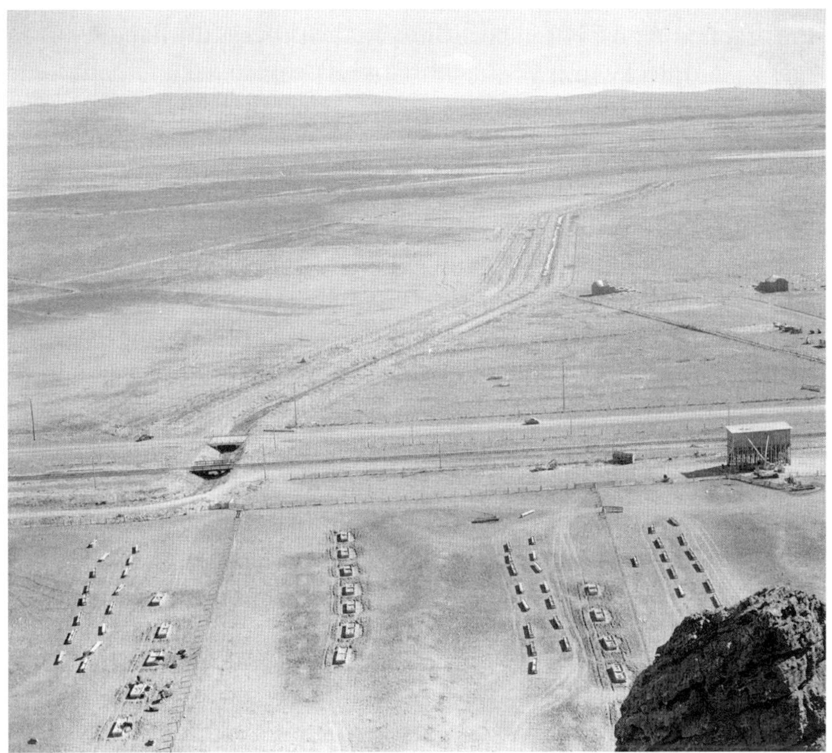

Tule Lake Relocation Center.

home so he could be with his wife, our mom. They finally said okay, and they released him. Two months before she died."

EMI (SOMEKAWA) BECKWITH

From Tule Lake, Emi and her family were transferred to Minidoka Relocation Center in Idaho. As in Heart Mountain, where many of the Nikkei medical staff staged a walkout over poor conditions, relationships between the European American and Nikkei medical staff were strained. Some of the white nurses were perceived as "just floating around and not working. Here they're getting high wages, and we worked like slaves with nothing."

Again, supplies and equipment were limited. As laundry facilities were insufficient, patients' linens were not changed every day as was the practice in hospitals before the war. “If it’s every third day, you’re lucky,” said Beckwith.

“And then your trays, your meal trays come in late, and sometimes your trays are there for a whole afternoon without being collected. There were a lot of things that just didn’t get done. There’s no one to blame.”

While in Minidoka, Beckwith’s family experienced personal tragedy. Her father-in-law, suffering from multiple strokes, finally died. Her aunt had been diagnosed with cervical cancer, and had even consulted with a doctor in Salt Lake City. But there was no effective treatment. “There was no use in keeping her in the hospital,” said Beckwith. “So we kept her in the barrack right next door to us. It was just plyboard that separated us, and you could hear everything that [went] on. She was just groaning and moaning.” To lessen her aunt’s pain, Emi was directed to give her a quarter grain of morphine about every two hours. Her aunt finally succumbed to cancer, leaving seven children in the care of her husband.

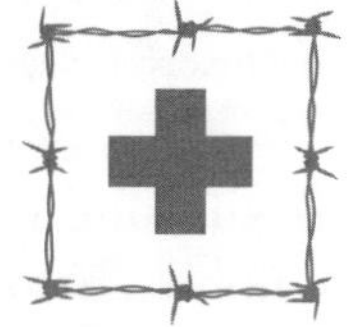

14. RESETTLEMENT AND RETURN TO THE WEST COAST

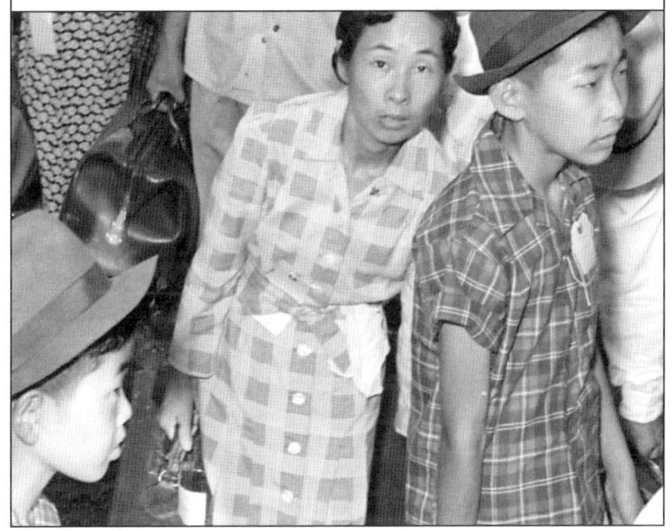

... if it weren't for the Japanese Hospital when I came back, I couldn't have done anything because [there was] *no hospital to work in.*

—Sakaye Shigekawa, MD, regarding her return to Los Angeles

Exclusion orders were rescinded in December 1944, enabling Japanese Americans to move back to the West Coast. Their return was not always welcomed. Tents, trailer parks, and hostels served as transitional housing. Many Japanese American doctors, for either family and professional reasons, decided to establish their practices in Japantowns or other communities where many Japanese American lived or worked.

HOMER YASUI

The former "impetuous boy" in Tule Lake Relocation Center, Homer Yasui had settled down in Colorado and completed his premed studies within three years at the University of Denver. It was August 1945, the official end of World War II, and time for Yasui to apply to medical school. He wrote to his father Masuo, who still remained incarcerated at Santa Fe alien detention center, that he applied to fifty schools, including two African American schools. One responded that "this is a medical school for black students only." Yasui received only one acceptance letter–from Hahnemann Medical in Philadelphia.

"You don't want to go to that school. That school's on probation," his advisor Humphrey Owens told him.

"What does that mean?" asked Yasui.

"It means it's not an up-and-up medical school, and if you graduate from there, you may not be recognized or get licensed."

"Well, Dr. Owens," replied Yasui, "it's the only one that accepted me."

Owens said that he didn't advise it, but Yasui felt that he had no other choice. He didn't want to "spin my wheels trying again next year."

"So I went and indeed Hahnemann was under probation that year because of the academic failings of the students," said Yasui. But in time Yasui's class excelled, enabling the reversal of the school's probationary status. "So I like to pride myself and say, 'Well, it was my class that pulled Hahnemann out of the academic doldrums, and it was reinstated to full glory and honor again.'"

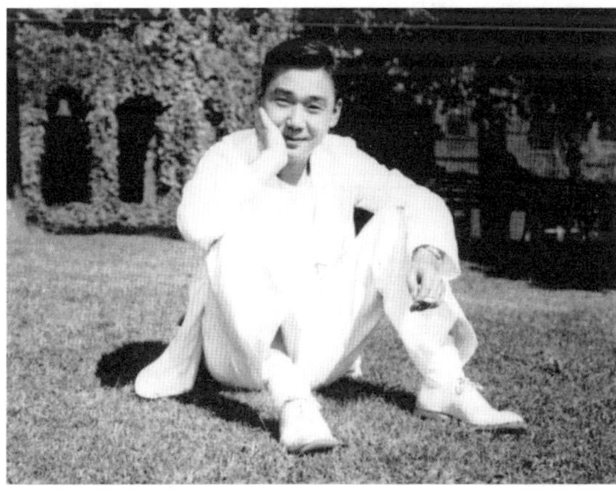

Dr. Homer Yasui in white intern's uniform, sitting on the back lawn of Vassar Brothers Hospital, Poughkeepsie, New York, 1951.

Of Yasui's classmates 10 percent were women, and 10 percent were Jewish Americans. In spite of these figures, Yasui did experience some incidents of discrimination while at Hahnemann. He and another Nisei, Bob Katase, had been invited to join a local medical fraternity. Then came an opportunity for the local to be recognized by the national organization.

"You know we want to affiliate," their fraternity president and brothers told them. "But they won't allow Japanese. So we'd like you guys to resign, quit. If you don't, we'll all quit."

"'Oh man,' I said, 'This is democratic?'

"And he said, 'Well, yes, that's democratic; I mean, majority rules.'

"So Bob and I resigned. So we never did become…national fraternity men."

The name of the national fraternity was Alpha Kappa Kappa. "They should have called it KKK, but they didn't," Yasui wryly observed.

WILLIAM SATO

William Sato, the only Asian American in his class at Northwestern Medical School in Illinois, also faced an incident of discrimination from a psychiatry professor. "He had all of us individually stand up and introduce ourselves: where we came from, and stuff like that. When it was my turn, I introduced myself and told them where I came from and then sat down.

"He made me stand up again, and he said, 'Wait a minute, now, what are you? Chinese or whatever?'

"I said, 'I'm an American of Japanese ancestry.'

"He said something that I couldn't get; my ears were still ringing [from the war] then. So I asked a fellow, because there was sort of a stir in the class.

"What did he say?" asked Sato.

His classmate said nothing. At the end of class, Sato went into the hallway and caught the attention of another student. "What did he say?" Sato asked again.

"No, Bill, you don't want to hear it."

"Yes, I do want to hear it."

Finally, the student relented. "The Professor said, 'We should have killed every goddamned one of you.'"

Later Sato confronted his professor, who was a German Jew. "With a name like yours, you had a lot of nerve saying what you did," said Sato, remembering his comrades who died in battle on the European front.

"Now, now, let's be nice," the professor replied.

"Why don't you be nice and apologize?" Sato retorted. But the professor turned and walked away. Sato did the same.

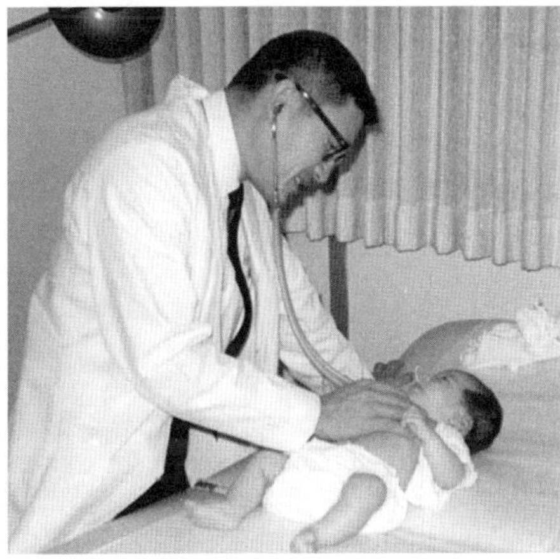
William Sato, MD, examining a young patient.

Now in hindsight, Sato said if he had heard the professor's remark during class, "it would have taken everything I had to keep from hitting him.... I've never forgiven myself for not doing something drastic."

After completing medical school, Dr. Sato interned at St. Luke's in Chicago followed by a surgical residency at West Suburban Hospital in Oak Park, Illinois, and was even offered an opportunity to join a general medical practice. But as the *chonan*, or oldest son, Dr. Sato thought that he and his family should return to Southern California, where his parents resided. But establishing his practice in the area where he spent his childhood proved difficult.

"We were still the pariahs in those days here on the West Coast. I couldn't lease an office space in a white building. They didn't want Japanese: 'We don't accept Japanese.'"

Sato first joined a practice with an established Nisei doctor, Dr. Norman Kobayashi, in the burgeoning Japanese American suburb of Gardena, located south of downtown Los Angeles. Investigating opportunities of opening his own office, he approached an European American pediatrician living in the Duarte-Monrovia area of East

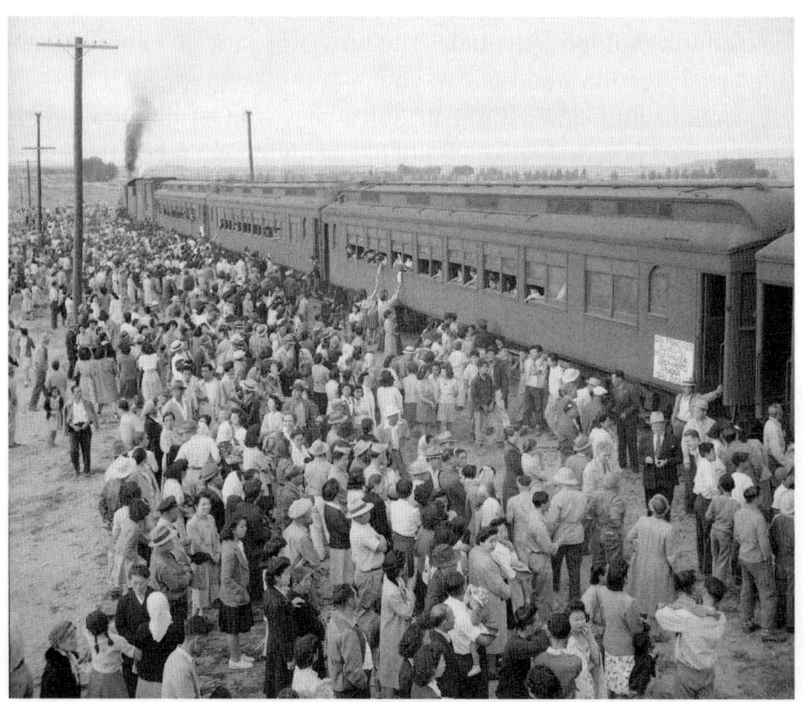

Incarcerees departing Heart Mountain Relocation Center.

San Gabriel Valley. “Why don’t you ask around and see if a Japanese American doctor could open up a practice in the area?” asked Sato. A couple of weeks later, the doctor returned with his reply: “You’re going to have a hard time if you try to open up a practice.”

That observation confirmed Sato’s initial impression: *I’ll have to deal with my own kind.* Even obtaining staff privileges was a challenge. “I tried to go to Good Samaritan here in the Los Angeles area, they wouldn’t accept me. . . . ‘We don’t want any Japanese.’ . . . [They] came right out and said that. So fortunately there was a little Japanese town here, an area called Little Tokyo, and we also had our Japanese Hospital.”

Dr. Hatsuji James Hara, who had been appointed the director of Los Angeles’ White Memorial Hospital in 1940, had made arrangements for this Seventh Day Adventist hospital to take care of the Japanese Hospital on Fickett Street during the war. In May 1946, the Japanese Hospital returned to Nikkei trusteeship.

Dr. Sato eventually opened up an office in a medical building just south of Los Angeles City Hall. He was not alone. Drawn to large numbers of Japanese American families living in the area, other Nisei doctors originally from Northern California and Washington state also established their practices in Los Angeles County in the 1950s. Regarding building up his patient load, Dr. Sato said, "For one, being with [Dr. Norman Kobayashi] in Gardena helped. Some of those people came with me; they would come [to Little Tokyo] and see me. Then my folks, I guess, pushed the word around. Also, I think I was able to put a little ad in the local vernacular, too, that I was opening a practice in such and such an area.

"It was an all-Japanese American practice. Even toward the end, it was mostly Japanese Americans."

SAKAYE SHIGEKAWA

Dr. Sakaye Shigekawa also felt fortunate that the Japanese Hospital was available for Nikkei doctors in Los Angeles: "If it weren't for the Japanese Hospital when I came back, I couldn't have done anything because [there was] no hospital to work in." Shigekawa had returned to Southern California from Chicago and in August 1949, purchased property on Santa Monica Boulevard in Los Angeles to start her own practice, which included obstetrics. Two area hospitals–Hollywood Presbyterian and Good Samaritan–refused to accept Japanese American doctors. Queen of Angels Hospital took a long time in responding, but finally after six months extended admitting privileges to both Shigekawa and an African American physician, a first in the history of the medical facility.

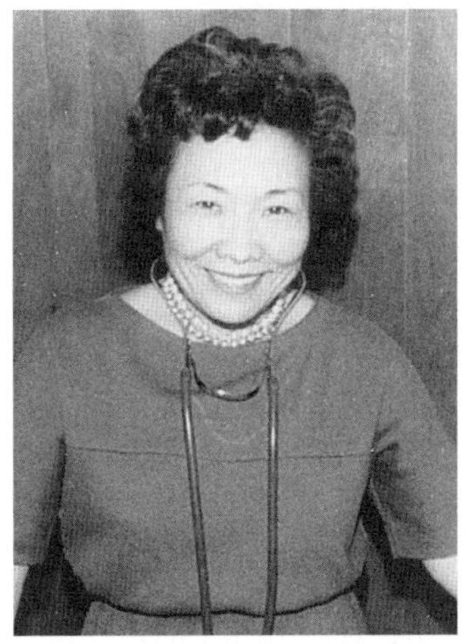

Dr. Sakaye Shigekawa at work.

However, even with Queen of Angels' more progressive policy, there were still problems. For instance, all of Shigekawa's patients were assigned to more expensive private rooms, while white patients were placed in four-bed wards, usually for five days to one week.

"Why is it that you send your patients home so early?" one of the nuns asked.

"Well, I didn't see why they should pay the penalty of being Japanese and not being put in the four-room wards," Shigekawa replied. She had heard that a supervising nun had declared that she would never mix the races in a hospital ward.

Shigekawa, however, had the support of one of the European American doctors. "I think you should mix them," he said. And finally, the integration process began at Queen of Angels Hospital in Los Angeles.

It has taken Shigekawa many years to speak candidly of her experience at Santa Anita Assembly Center. "The minute I'd talk about it, I was crying. I couldn't talk about it. Now I can talk about it pretty freely, but I couldn't, because [of] the way they took away some of the parents, and they didn't know where they were going to be. The family didn't know what to do. None of that is ever told. They'd be walking down someplace, and... the FBI would yank them out, and the families didn't see them again. I know my father had the hog ranch in Long Beach, and on the way home, he was taken and jailed for a day, too.... Then the way that, when we were in camp... [and they] were returned home, and you saw them, just broken-down people. Men that were very vivacious and very energetic, all of a sudden, they were old men in less than six months. Some had had strokes in the meantime.

"All these things, you know, that happened, I just couldn't talk about it. It was so depressing, and so... so cruel. So I just couldn't talk about it."

Shigekawa cites her work experience with doctors such as Dr. Norman Kobayashi and Dr. Fred Fujikawa as her salvation during those depressing months in Santa Anita Assembly Center. "They helped me see the light, accept the situation, and make the best of it. So then I was so busy seeing patients. As I say, if it weren't for my career, I think I would have been a very, very unhappy person."

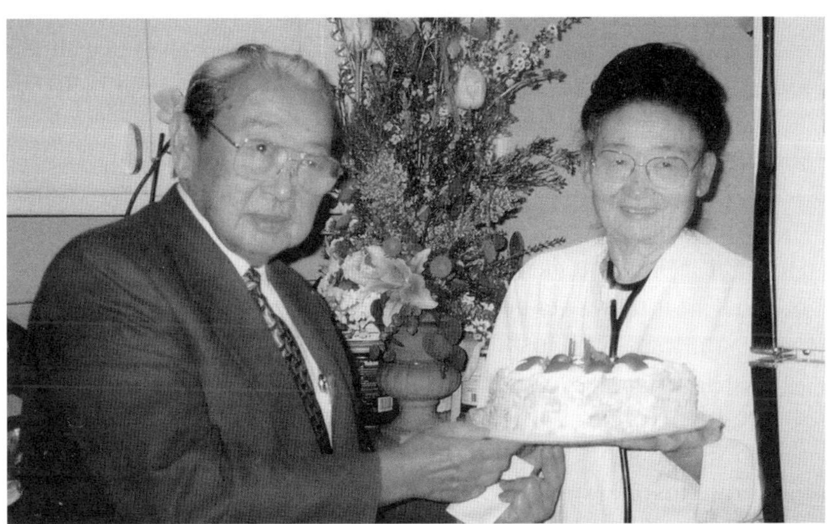

Drs. Sanbo S. Sakaguchi and Mary Sakaguchi Oda, at Dr. Oda's 80th birthday party in their San Fernando office, March 2000.

SANBO SAKAGUCHI
MARY SAKAGUCHI ODA

Completing two years of thoracic surgery residency in Milwaukee, Dr. Sanbo Sakaguchi moved to the San Fernando Valley in Southern California, where his older brother Chibo was practicing dentistry. During his first year of practice, Sakaguchi assisted Dr. James Goto, who had returned to Southern California after the war. "He was a few years older than I was, and he had a tremendous practice. He was trained in general surgery, but he did general practice. He was one of the big practitioners in Little Tokyo."

In February 1950, Sakaguchi borrowed $10,000 from a bank to open his own office. "I had to buy a lot of equipment and everything. I first had my office on San Fernando Road and Maclay, on the second floor. It was an old office [of] a doctor [who] had built a new office so that was open. I decided I'll just start... I decided that I'll just do general practice and then do surgery, because in those days, most of the doctors were all general practitioners. They did everything. They did deliveries. They did surgery."

What proved to be a larger problem was finding a facility that would grant him hospital privileges. "In the valley here, there [were] three hospitals. One was San Fernando Hospital–that was a small community hospital, and in the bylaws, it stated that if you practiced in the city of San Fernando, you automatically become a member of the hospital staff." The two other hospitals, however, did not even acknowledge Sakaguchi's application. "They just ignored me. Well, I didn't have that many hospital patients. But then there was a Japanese Hospital at First and Fickett in Los Angeles. So I got on the staff there, but that's a long way to go, twenty-three miles into Los Angeles."

As San Fernando Hospital was the closest facility for his patients, Sakaguchi ended up sending most of them there. Then he was drafted during the Korean War but received a deferment for three years, thereby missing the conflict. He went on to serve two years at Madigan General Hospital near Tacoma, Washington, and returned to private practice in 1955.

In 1960, Sakaguchi's younger sister, Dr. Mary Oda, joined the practice. After leaving Manzanar, Oda had completed her education and internship at Women's Medical College in Philadelphia. "We were in a clinic," Oda said regarding her experience in Philadelphia, "and the professor said, 'Examine this woman and tell me what's wrong with her.'

"So I examined her. In those days, we had no CAT scans. All we had were X-rays. We had no CAT scans, no MRIs, nothing. We had to go by what we could hear with our stethoscopes and percussion.

"So I percussed her chest, and he said, 'What's wrong with this lady?'

"I was the only one, I said, 'She's got amphoric resonance. She's got a cavity.' And I was right. (Tuberculosis was often a cause of such pulmonary cavity formation.)

"I think the professor was impressed because I was the only one that knew anything about amphoric resonance, because I had read that book when I was in camp. Then I had gotten so I could pick up murmurs. To this day, I pick up murmurs that cardiologists miss because I spent a year and a half just listening to murmurs, listening to lungs, examining patients. So that's the only thing positive I got out of camp, is I learned to listen to hearts and lungs."

AUGUSTUS "GUS" TANAKA
BENJAMIN TANAKA

When Dr. Benjamin Tanaka was finally released from Santa Fe alien detention center, he headed straight for Salt Lake City to be reunited with his wife who was working as a live-in domestic. Together they went back to Portland, where the reaction to returning Japanese Americans was less than welcoming. As his son Gus reported, "He was pretty much told that he couldn't get on the staff of the hospital any more there.... He had been on the staff of those two hospitals, and they said there was no room for him there. He didn't have a location to practice and so forth. At the same time, the people here were ready to find him a place. He needed to borrow money, which I think he did from some of his friends here, to get started."

The new start was in Ontario, a city in eastern Oregon on the Idaho border well outside the military areas. Before the war, approximately 134 Japanese Americans lived in Ontario and its surrounding Malheur County. As reported by Florangela Davila, that population quickly grew to one thousand as Malheur County, designated a "free zone" open to individuals of Japanese ancestry, recruited farm workers during World War II. Ontario's mayor, Elmo Smith, also publisher of the *Eastern Observer* newspaper, agreed to host Japanese Americans: "If the Japs, both alien and nationals, are a menace to the Pacific Coast safety unless they are moved inland," he said to the Associated Press, "it appears downright cowardly to take any other stand than to put out the call, 'Send them along; we'll cooperate to the fullest possible extent in taking care of them.'"

After the war, some families chose to stay. They would become Dr. Benjamin Tanaka's patients. "He felt that this was a much friendlier place, and he went up to talk to the nuns here at the [Holy Rosary] Hospital. They just threw their arms right open and welcomed him with open arms," said Gus.

Meanwhile, Gus had returned to Haverford College in Pennsylvania to complete his undergraduate work. He then applied to medical schools, but with the large number of returning soldiers like himself, he knew that competition would be tough. "... I knew that there was a backlog of applicants because there were a lot of GIs that didn't get into medical school because they were drafted or reserved. I also knew that there were a lot of GIs that started looking at medicine as a possible career because with the GI bill they could afford something that they would not have given much thought to. My decision was to grab the first acceptance that came along."

The first school to accept Gus was the Long Island College of Medicine in Brooklyn (now known as the State University of New York). He earned his medical degree with honors in 1951. Seven years later, he completed his surgical residency at Kings County Hospital, associated with SUNY Medical School. After spending nearly a decade on the East Coast, Gus was now being called back to Oregon and specifically to his father's practice in the town of Ontario.

"My dad had written a number of times, strongly hinting that he'd like to have me come back. The hinting got to the point where he was almost saying, 'I need you.' While I was in training, I seriously considered staying in academic medicine. There were some things about academic medicine that disenchanted me... I saw evidence of [a] kind of competitiveness, which was less than cordial—cutthroat, publish or perish, and those kinds of things, which I thought I could live my life without.

"When Dad approached me the way he did, it gave me an opportunity perhaps to pay back for the opportunity that he was able to provide me in being able to get to where I had gotten."

On January 2, 1959, father and son opened the Tanaka Clinic in Ontario. The practice grew to include six physicians. From the very beginning, Gus did not feel confined by the farm community he was serving. "...The world, when you're working, is only what you see immediately around you," said Gus. "So the size of the community itself didn't bother me, as long as there was enough stuff to keep me busy. I found that there was more than enough to keep me busy when I was in practice there."

His father, Dr. Benjamin Tanaka, continued to practice on a gradually reduced workload until he was about eighty-four years old. He died in 1975, one month shy of his eighty-eighth birthday. "But my dad...felt that he had a good life here in this country in spite of everything," said Gus, who retired in 1993. "People have asked him about bitterness and so forth. And he said, yes, he would have his moments of anger about all of this, and he felt a little bit piqued about the fact that people in effect would hold him responsible for the war... when he had nothing to do with it, and didn't sympathize with it. But he figured the treatment the Japanese got here was really an aberration of fundamental American principles, and it would work itself out, and it did. It has."

TOGASAKI SISTERS

Only two of the Togasaki sisters—Kazue and Yoshiye—returned to their hometown, the San Francisco Bay Area, to practice medicine. Regarding their legacy to their other family members, nephew Gordon Togasaki said, "I think it's the compassion for all human beings. I think I could summarize it just there. A tremendous amount of compassion, empathy. When the chips were down, economics were not a problem. They just did what they thought was right. And they had to fight through the most difficult time for women. Each one had to fight and was a trailblazer. In terms of Yoshiye and public health, the men just blocked her. They wouldn't make her commissioner.

"So there has been a period, not because you're Japanese American or Japanese, it's just between female and male. They were female doctors in a period where they had to break through the barriers.... So for us we kind of look back and say, 'What did they leave to us?' Basically it's that we just got to return, in our own way... to society.... I think that's the kind of legacy that we have inherited. I don't know if that will continue with the next generation or not, but for me that's [it]. I was watching what they did....

"[Once] I said, 'I don't know how we're going to be able to repay you for all you did for us.'

"[Kazue] looked after me when I came home from school, and Yoshiye looked after my sister.

"Her one comment was, 'We won't be here. Just do the same thing for somebody else down the line....'

"So that pretty much speaks for her. But we can't possibly meet what they've done. It's just too much."

GEORGE TARO AKAMATSU

In August 1945, Dr. George Akamatsu's cousin brought a used car to Minidoka Relocation Center so that Akamatsu and his wife Yasuka could return to the West Coast. Reestablishing a practice in Walnut Grove, once a thriving Japanese community, was out of the question. Most of the former Walnut Grove residents had scattered throughout the United States to Denver, Chicago, and Minnesota. Instead, they aimed for the next best thing: Sacramento.

Yasuka Akamatsu reported: "As soon as we returned to Sacramento, California, [he] rented a couple of rooms in a hotel and started practicing medicine. He had to purchase new medical equipment and furniture. This was a temporary office until he found a suitable office. A few months later, he moved into an office in the downtown area. Several years later, the city redevelopment program took over the area so he had to move again. He found a place closer to home and practiced medicine until December 1, 1967. He suffered a stroke and passed away on January 12, 1968.

"He liked children because we didn't have any. He just loved them, especially little girls. After we came back to Sacramento, we'd go to the Japanese Methodist church here. All those girls that he delivered, they became teenagers.

"They'd all pass by and say, 'Hi, Doc!' 'Hi, Doc!' And they won't say hi to me.

"I just kidded the girls, 'You pass by me and say, 'Hi, Doc.'

"'Oh,' one of the girls said, 'he [is] our favorite doctor.'"

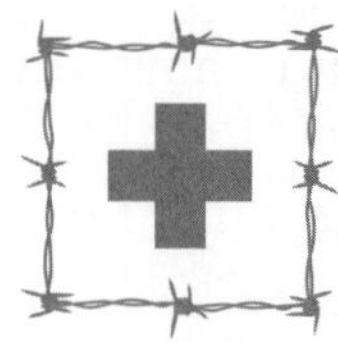

EPILOGUE

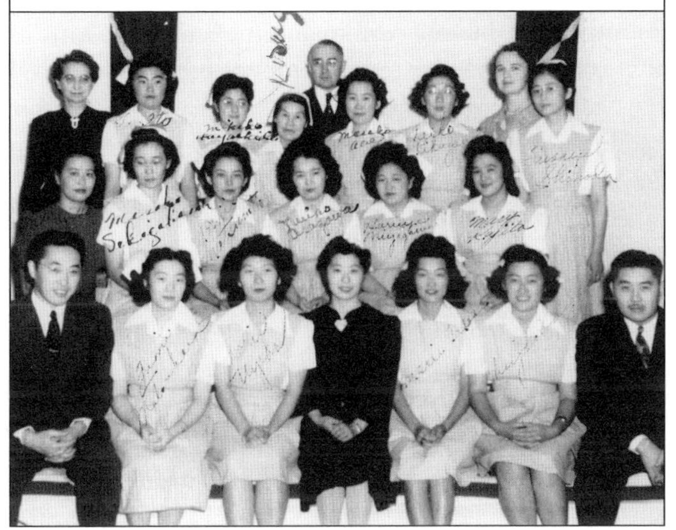

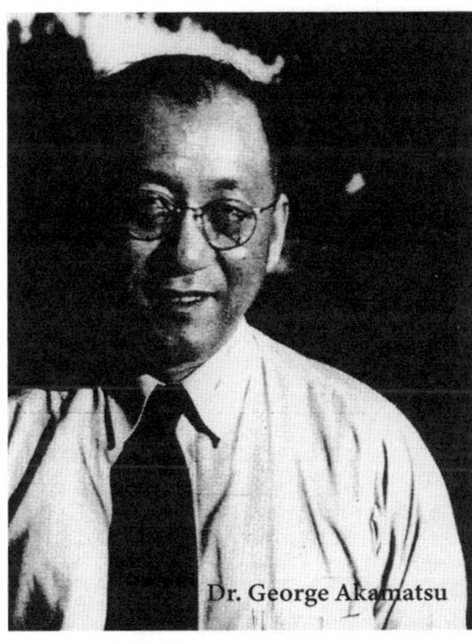
Dr. George Akamatsu

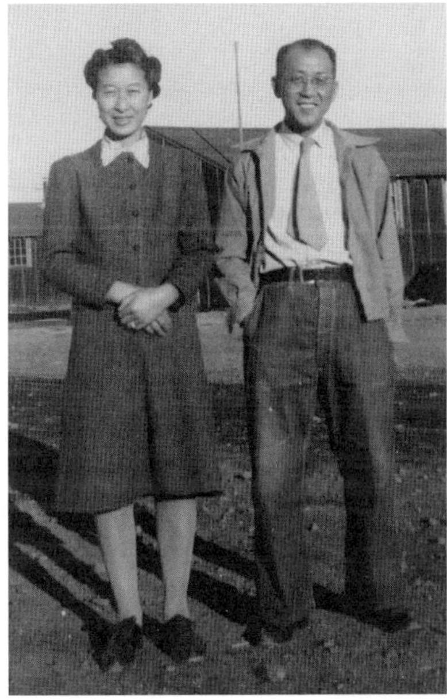

AKAMATSU, Dr. George Taro

FAMILY PRACTICE PHYSICIAN

b. 1899 Momoshima,
Hiroshima-ken, Japan
d. 1968 Sacramento, CA

1936 MD, Emory School of Medicine, Decatur, GA
1937 Internship, Columbus City Hospital, Columbus, GA
1938 Set up practice in Walnut Grove, CA
1942 Puyallup Assembly Center, Tule Lake, Minidoka, physician

Before the war, **Dr. George Akamatsu** practiced medicine in Walnut Grove, California. When the Akamatsus married in Seattle in 1930, his wife Yasuka lost her U.S. citizenship because she married a non-citizen. Ironically, if they had waited one year, the law was amended and she could have retained her rights. Seven years later she regained her citizenship. Dr. Akamatsu began seeing patients in Sacramento soon after his return from incarceration in 1945. One of his happiest days came on March 2, 1953, when he received his U.S. citizenship. An avid fisherman, he and his wife spent many Wednesdays fishing around the Sacramento area. He practiced medicine until December 1, 1967, when he suffered a stroke. He was hospitalized until his death on January 12, 1968.

PAUL TSUNEISHI interviewed Yasuka Akamatsu on November 26, 2002, in Sacramento, CA, about the life of her husband.

BABA, Dr. George Ryoji

OBSTETRICIAN/GYNECOLOGIST
b. 1913 San Francisco, CA
d. 1995 Santa Clara, CA

1938 MD, University of California Medical School, San Francisco, CA
1942 Turlock Assembly Center, Gila River, Tule Lake, physician
1943 Residency OB/GYN, Chicago, IL

Dr. George Baba's medical experience prior to World War II included earning his MD from the University of California Medical School, a two-year OB/GYN internship, and one year at St. Luke's Hospital in Japan. He had two years of private practice in San Francisco before the war and incarceration disrupted his life. Dr. Baba helped vaccinate people in San Francisco who were leaving for Tanforan Assembly Center, a racetrack in San Bruno, California. But because there were not enough physicians in the San Joaquin Valley, he was sent to Turlock Assembly Center and then on to Gila River. From there he was transferred to Tule Lake. In April 1943, he left Tule Lake for a five-year OB/GYN residency in Chicago. After the war, Dr. Baba set up an obstetrics and gynecological practice in Little Tokyo, downtown Los Angeles. Later, he moved to Santa Clara, California.

The Japanese American Medical Association and the Japanese American National Museum are the recipients of Dr. Baba's medical papers and memorabilia, courtesy of Mrs. Baba.

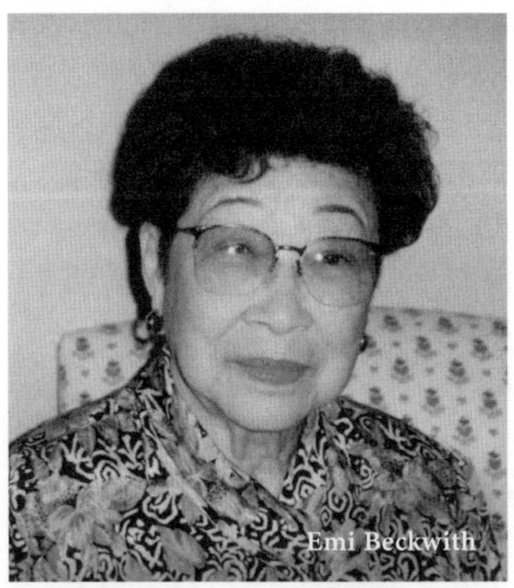
Emi Beckwith

BECKWITH, Emi Somekawa

REGISTERED NURSE
b. 1918 Portland, OR
d. 2020 Puyallup, WA

1939: RN, Emanuel Hospital, Portland, OR
1942: Portland Assembly Center, Tule Lake, Minidoka, registered nurse

Emi Somekawa and her husband Arthur left Minidoka for jobs in the Midwest. He found work in an Indiana steel factory but developed lead poisoning. She worked as a nurse for a farm labor camp and later for the Sioux Ordinance Depot in Nebraska. While there, Arthur joined her until they were able to return to Portland where the Somekawas found renters had left their house unlivable. The emotional strain of resettlement caused Emi to develop a six-month case of hives. Promised her old job back, she returned to Emanuel Hospital and was rehired as supervisor of the labor and delivery room. After their two children were in college, she found it difficult to mesh hospital hours with her husband's work schedule so she quit and went to work more regular hours in a doctor's office. When her husband was transferred to Auburn, Washington, in 1955, the couple moved to Puyallup where Emi worked for several doctors until she retired at age sixty-two. She continued working part-time and later took a job cooking for a Red Cross Issei senior citizen's program. Her husband passed away in 1978, and she married an old family friend, Vance Beckwith, in 1997.

GWENN M. JENSEN interviewed Mrs. Beckwith on July 22, 2002, in Puyallup, Washington.

CHUMAN, Frank F.

ATTORNEY
b. 1917 Montecito, CA

1942: Manzanar, hospital administrator
1945: JD, University of Maryland School of Law, Baltimore, MD

Mr. Frank F. Chuman, an attorney, graduated from UCLA in 1938 and attended law school at USC from 1940 to 1942. After he left Manzanar, he completed his law school training at the University of Maryland. Upon his return to Los Angeles, he went to work for the law firm that served as counsel for the ACLU. He soon opened his own private practice and specialized in immigration law. Active in many community organizations, he also served as national president of the Japanese American Citizens League (JACL) from 1960 to 1962. Seven years of research and writing resulted in his book, *The Bamboo People: The Law and Japanese-Americans* published in 1976. The volume is a legal history of people of Japanese ancestry from the first immigrant to America in the 1880s through 1965. Nearly thirty years later, the book is still hailed as "authoritative" and "provocative." Mr. Chuman is well known in professional law circles and for his work on behalf of the Japanese American community. The foundation he created funds scholarships for law students. In 2000, he moved to Thailand with his wife, Donna.

NAOMI HIRAHARA interviewed Mr. Chuman on November 21, 2002, in Los Angeles, CA.

FUJIKAWA, Dr. Yoshihiko Fred

THORACIC SURGEON & PULMONOLOGIST
b. 1910 San Francisco, CA
d. 1992 Seal Beach, CA

1934: MD, Creighton University School of Medicine, Omaha, NE
1936: Two-year internship, L.A. County General Hospital, Los Angeles, CA
1942: Santa Anita Assembly Center, Jerome, physician

After he received his medical training, **Dr. Fred Fujikawa** opened a private practice on Terminal Island, California. Six years later, he and his wife Alice were one of the first people of Japanese ancestry to be incarcerated in Santa Anita. In November of 1943, with his family, he departed

Jerome Relocation Center for a residency in thoracic medicine at the Missouri State Sanatorium in Mount Vernon. While there, he became the target of an unsuccessful legislative attempt to ban "non-state" physicians from practicing in Missouri. As this furor raged in the state legislature and local newspapers, Dr. Fujikawa continued to treat patients at the sanatorium. In 1946, he was named a fellow of the American College of Chest Physicians, and in 1948, a fellow of the American College of Surgeons. The Fujikawas returned to Southern California with their three children in 1949, and he opened offices in Little Tokyo and Long Beach where he treated pulmonary diseases and did thoracic surgery. In recognition of a seminal paper on pulmonary tuberculosis presented at a chest conference in Tokyo, Fujikawa became the first foreigner to receive a Doctorate of Medical Science degree from Keio University. He retired from surgery in 1975 and volunteered his time with TB patients at the chest clinic of the Long Beach City Health Department.

Naomi Hirahara interviewed Dr. Fujikawa for Japanese Community Health, Inc. on April 1, 1989, in Seal Beach, California.

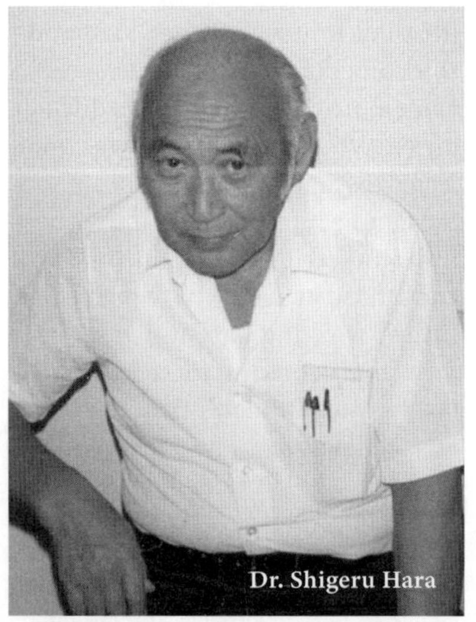
Dr. Shigeru Hara

HARA, Dr. Shigeru

GENERAL PRACTITIONER
b. 1911 Sacramento, CA
d. 2004 San Diego, CA

1941 MD, Marquette School of Medicine, Milwaukee, WI
Internship started at Sacramento County Hospital, Sacramento, CA
1942 Marysville (Arboga) Assembly Center, Tule Lake, physician
1943 Volunteered for U.S. Army, Carlisle Barracks, PA, Camp Shelby, MS, Sixth Army, TX and MA
1944 Camp Miami, Reims, France

Dr. Shig Hara volunteered for the service so he could become an officer rather than be drafted as a private. As he left Tule Lake in his first lieutenant's uniform, the guards saluted him on his way out, much to the delight of the girls in the hospital. A workhorse, he requested ward duty for his military assignment, overseeing as many as eight wards at a time. While overseas, he treated many of the GIs for malaria, which they had contracted fighting in Italy. Upon his return from his European tour of duty in January 1945, he learned his brother George had established a dental practice in San Diego and invited him to join him there. With his wife Lorraine and their two children, Glen and Susan, Dr. Hara moved to San Diego and opened his practice in 1946. After his wife of twenty-five years passed away, he married Connie, his office nurse, five years later. He retired at the age of eighty, having practiced medicine for more than fifty years and delivering several thousand babies.

GWENN M. JENSEN interviewed Dr. Hara on December 4, 2002, in San Diego, California.

KAMBARA, Dr. George K.

OPHTHALMOLOGIST
b. 1916 Sacramento, CA
d. 2001 Los Angeles, CA

1941 MD, Stanford University School of Medicine, San Francisco, CA
Surgical Internship, one-year rotating, Stanford-Lane Hospitals, San Francisco, CA
1942 Began ENT residency, Stanford-Lane Hospitals, San Francisco, CA
Marysville (Arboga) Assembly Center, Tule Lake, physician

Dr. George Kambara started a residency in ear, nose, and throat (ENT) at Stanford because he could not afford the application fees for L.A. County General Hospital, his first choice. His resident's salary of $25 per month afforded him enough income to marry May Tanaka, a registered nurse. He resigned his position on March 26, 1942, and moved to Sacramento so that he could be sent to the same center as his parents. In 1943, he left Tule Lake for an eye, ear, nose, throat (EENT) residency at the Memphis Eye, Ear, Nose, and Throat Hospital in Tennessee. While completing this eighteen-month rotation, however, he decided ophthalmology was more interesting. Since his ENT training was not sufficient for board certification, he took an additional year of an ophthalmology residency at the State of Wisconsin General Hospital in Madison. The Kambaras returned to California in June 1948. Although initially he had trouble finding office space, he established his own practice in central Los Angeles and was accepted to the staff of White Memorial Hospital. Eventually, he became chief of the eye service at White Memorial and Rancho Los Amigos Hospital in Downey. He taught at Loma Linda University, the University of California at Irvine, and the University of Southern California. Dr. Kambara retired in 1983, after caring for thousands of patients and two generations of medical residents.

Dr. Kambara's widow, May, donated his medical correspondence and memorabilia to JAMA and the Japanese American National Museum.

KAWAKAMI, Dr. Iwao George

GENERAL SURGEON
b. 1921 Los Angeles, CA
d. 2024 Los Angeles, CA

1942 Santa Anita Assembly Center, ambulance driver and orderly, Gila River, medical statistician
1944 Drafted into U.S. Army, Jefferson Barracks, MO, Camp Maxey, TX
1945 Medic, Occupation of Italy
1951 MD, University of Rochester School of Medicine, Rochester, NY

Although **Dr. Iwao Kawakami** served in the postwar occupation of Italy, conflict still raged between Italy and Yugoslavia and his unit came under fire many times. His assignment was as a medic for a tank battalion. After his discharge, he was grateful to have the GI Bill to pay for his medical education as his father had lost his store when they were incarcerated and had to start over, working as a gardener at age sixty. When Dr. Kawakami received his MD from the University of Rochester in 1951, he decided to stay in Rochester while he completed a five-year surgical residence at Genesee Hospital. He married Toyoko Kitajima in 1953, and they set up housekeeping on his $15-a-month resident's salary. When he returned to Los Angeles in 1956, he became a research surgeon working on coronary artery disease in the dog laboratory at UCLA. At the same time, he opened his private surgical practice in Mar Vista, a nearby community. After seven years, he left UCLA and devoted himself full-time to his private practice. In 1993, Dr. Kawakami stopped doing surgery and two years later retired completely at the age of seventy-four.

GWENN M. JENSEN interviewed Dr. Kawakami on August 15, 2002, in Los Angeles, California.

KINOSHITA, Dr. Robert S.

FAMILY PRACTITIONER & SURGEON
b. 1906 Honolulu, HI
d. 2001 Gresham, OR

1934 MD, University of Nebraska College of Medicine, Omaha, NE
1935 Internship, Emanuel Hospital, Portland, OR
Contract physician (Army), Civilian Conservation Corps
1939 District surgeon (Army), Medford District CCC, OR
1942 Portland Assembly Center, Heart Mountain, physician
1943 Volunteered U.S. Army 442d Regimental Combat Team, Camp McCoy, WI, Camp Shelby, MS, Seventh Armored Division, Ft. Benning, GA
1944 Battalion Surgeon, Overseas with Seventh Armored and 102nd Infantry.
Received Silver Star/Oak Leaf Cluster, Bronze Star/OLC, and Purple Heart/2 OLC, Combat Medic Badge

Dr. Robert Kinoshita returned from Europe in 1945, and worked at the Percy Jones Military Hospital in Battle Creek, Michigan, until his discharge from the Army in June 1946. He returned to Portland, Oregon, with his wife and two sons, where he set up a private practice. Initially he was unable to obtain hospital privileges, but with the help of physicians who knew him before the war and an article that appeared in *The Oregonian* about his exemplary military career, doors finally opened in 1947. The incarceration adversely affected both his and his wife's health. He developed gastrointestinal problems at Heart Mountain, which eventually became bleeding stomach ulcers while he was training medics for the 442d RCT. His health worsened when he returned to Portland with the stress of starting over in a hostile environment. Because of his condition and his wife's poor health, he had to turn down an offer from the Army to attend Staff College, an advance to the rank of lieutenant colonel, and any future command positions, which for him was the job of his dreams. In spite of his affliction, he maintained a full practice but eventually underwent a subtotal gastrectomy. He continued seeing patients until his retirement in 1976. He, along with his wife Evelyn, a registered nurse, were honored in 1996, for service to the Medford District of the CCC and nearby civilian communities in the Umpqua Valley, Oregon. Dr. Kinoshita died on January 2, 2001, followed five days later by his wife of more than sixty years.

GWENN M. JENSEN interviewed Dr. Kinoshita's son Richard about the life of his father on July 24, 2002, in Portland, Oregon.

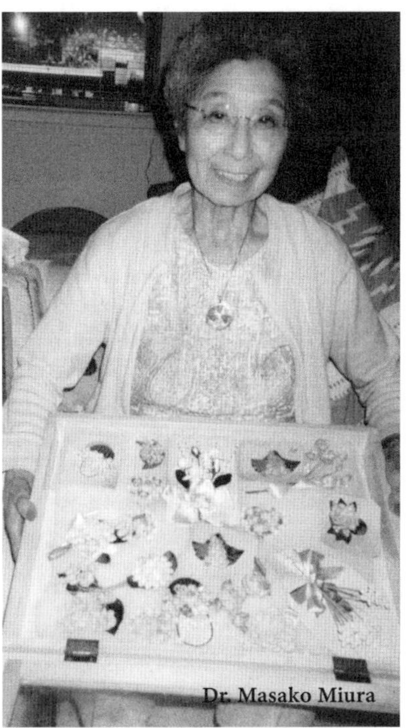

Dr. Masako Miura

MIURA, Dr. Masako (Kusayanagi)

DERMATOLOGIST
b. 1914 Pasadena, CA
d. 2023 Watsonville, CA

1941 MD, University of Southern California School of Medicine, Los Angeles, CA
Internship, St. Anthony's Hospital, Terre Haute, IN
Began three-year syphilology and dermatology residency, L.A. County General Hospital, Los Angeles, CA
1942 Manzanar, physician
1943 Topaz, physician

Upon her return from Topaz, **Dr. Masako (Kusayanagi) Miura** applied for reinstatement to her residency at

L.A. County General Hospital within the required ninety-day period. At first, the County Commissioners said, "This is not the propitious time." However, when she told them she expected to hear from them when it was "propitious" or they would hear from her lawyer, they found an opening in the Dermatology Department. After her three-year residency, she joined her husband, Dr. Goto, in his practice in her father's building for a few years. Next she went to work for the L.A. County School System as a school physician from 1953 to 1955 and raised their daughter, Denise, and son, Hans. When her marriage ended, she moved to Oakland and joined the staff at Oakland Army Base Hospital. One year later she transferred to Fort Ord Hospital in Monterey where she married Kiyoshi Miura, an agricultural supply specialist, in 1955. They made their home in the Watsonville area. After almost thirty years of medical practice, she retired at the age of sixty-eight. Her husband passed away in 1994.

GWENN M. JENSEN interviewed Dr. Miura on September 2, 2002, in Aptos, California.

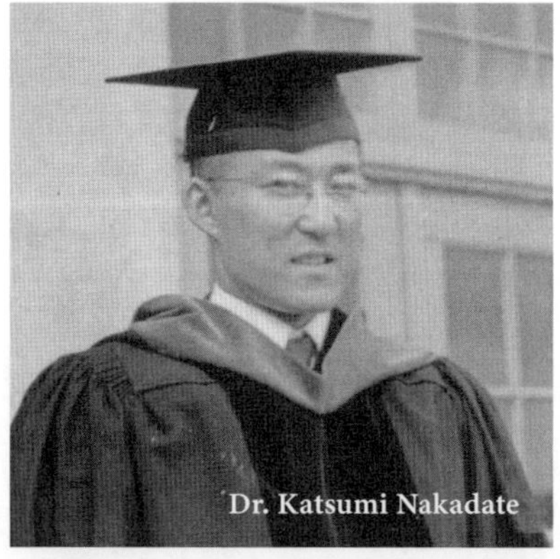
Dr. Katsumi Nakadate

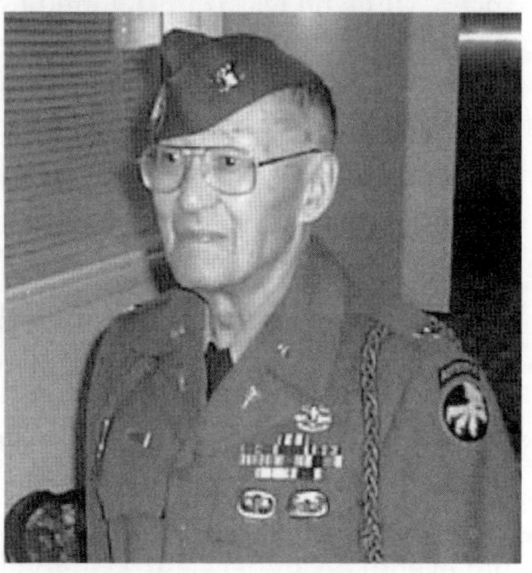

NAKADATE, Dr. Katsumi James

ANESTHESIOLOGIST
b. 1914 Portland, OR
d. 2007 Portland, OR

1939 MD, University of Oregon Medical School, Portland, OR
1940 Internship, St. Catherine's Hospital, East Chicago, IN
Began internal medicine residency, Eloise Hospital, Detroit, MI
1943 U.S. Army, trained 442d Regimental Combat Team medics

1944 Battalion Aid Station Doctor, Sixty-ninth Division, reassigned to Seventeenth and later the Eighty-second Airborne. Awarded Silver Star, Purple Heart.

After the war, **Dr. Katsumi James Nakadate** entered private practice. Because his war injuries limited his ability to get around, he decided to retrain in anesthesiology and attended the University of Illinois Research and Education Hospital in Chicago for two years while maintaining a working relationship with the local VA hospital. He went to work for Mercy Hospital in Gary, Indiana, for two years, where three of their four children were born, and then returned to the Pacific Northwest. A brief stint at the Veteran's Administration Hospital in Walla Walla, Washington, was followed by nearly twenty-five years of service at St. Vincent Hospital in Portland, Oregon, where he retired as chief anesthesiologist. Over the years, he retained his interest in Boy Scouting. His son Neil reports his father's favorite saying is, "Be prepared," especially where his patients or fishing were concerned. After his retirement in 1981, he volunteered at the Epworth Methodist Church Senior Center providing blood pressure checks and flu shots. His wife Mary passed away in 2000 after fifty-eight years of marriage.

GWENN M. JENSEN interviewed Dr. Nakadate on July 26, 2002, in Portland, Oregon.

OBI, Dr. Robert Toshio

ANESTHESIOLOGY, HOSPITAL MEDICAL DIRECTOR

b. 1918 Los Angeles, CA
d. 1999, South Pasadena, CA

1942 Santa Anita Assembly Center, hospital extern, Amache, chief X-ray technician

1948 MD, Wayne State University School of Medicine, Detroit, MI

Dr. Robert Obi started medical school at the University of Southern California in 1940, but midway through his second year, the war broke out, and he and his family were sent to Santa Anita. He left Amache in 1944, to work as a biochemist for the Children's Fund in Detroit, Michigan. Within four years of leaving Amache, he had obtained his medical degree from Wayne State University in Detroit. At that point, he chose to return to Los Angeles and did his internship and anesthesiology residency at L.A. County General Hospital. He went on to become Medical Director of the Japanese Hospital/City View Hospital and taught at USC Medical Center. When City View Hospital closed in 1985, Dr. Obi retired and devoted himself to service in the Japanese American community and was active in the Japanese American Citizens League, the Japanese Community Health, Inc., and the biennial Hiroshima Survivor's Clinic.

NAOMI HIRAHARA interviewed Dr. Obi for Japanese Community Health, Inc., on June 20, 1990, in South Pasadena, California.

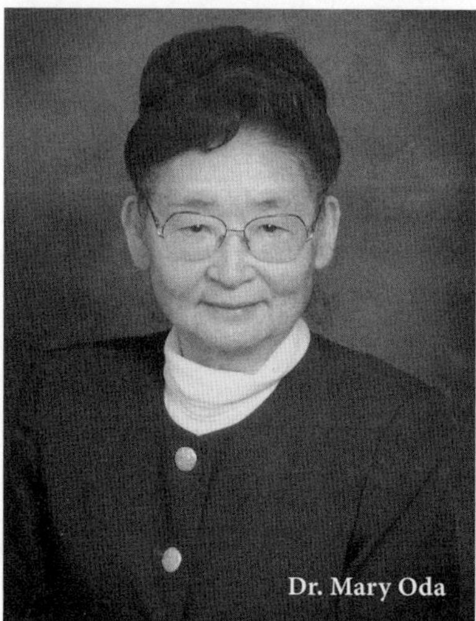
Dr. Mary Oda

ODA, Dr. Mary Sakaguchi

GENERAL PRACTITIONER
b. 1920, Fresno County, CA
d. 2013, Northridge, CA

1941 Medical student, University of California Medical School, San Francisco, CA
1942 Manzanar, phlebotomist, lab technician,
and physician's assistant
1946 MD, Women's Medical College (now MCP Hahnemann Medical School), Philadelphia, PA

While **Dr. Mary Sakaguchi Oda** was between her second and third year of medical school, she married her husband James whom she had met at Manzanar. Pregnant during her final year of medical school, she gave birth to their first daughter, Rosemarie, a month after graduating in 1946. When her husband James took a job as a translator and interpreter in Japan, Dr. Oda accepted what she describes as the hardest job of her life: she became a housewife for the next seven years. Upon their return to the States with their two daughters, she went to work for seven years at the state mental hospital in Pomona, now called Lanterman Developmental Center. During that time she gave birth to a third daughter, Maryjane, in 1952, and a son, Eugene in 1956. In 1959 she began a residency in psychiatry, but at the end of her first year of residency, her brother, Sanbo, invited her to join him in his practice in the San Fernando Valley.

GWENN M. JENSEN interviewed Dr. Oda on August 15, 2002, in San Fernando, California.

SAKAGUCHI, Dr. Sanbo

THORACIC SURGEON
b. 1917 Los Angeles, CA
d. 2013 Granada Hills, CA

1943 MD, Marquette School of Medicine, Milwaukee, WI
1944 General surgery internship, Milwaukee County General Hospital, WI
1947 General surgery residency, Milwaukee County General Hospital, WI
1949 Thoracic surgery residency, Milwaukee County and Muirdale Sanitarium, WI

When **Dr. Sanbo Sakaguchi** graduated with his MD in 1943, he got a call from the procurement and assignment headquarters of the U.S. Army wanting to know his classification. When he told them 4-C, he never heard from them again. He completed

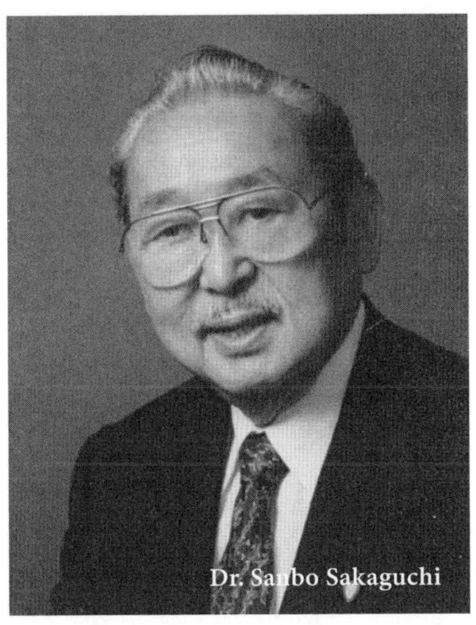
Dr. Sanbo Sakaguchi

his two residencies in surgery in 1949, returned to Los Angeles, and joined his older brother, Chebo, who had a dental office in San Fernando. Shortly after starting his private practice, his Selective Service classification changed from 4-C to 1-A, and he was drafted. He applied for a deferment on the grounds that he was the only Japanese-speaking doctor in San Fernando and received a three-year extension. Before he heard from the army again, he married Kay Furuta in 1952, and when the time came, he reported to Fort Sam Houston for basic training. He received orders to report to Madigan General Hospital near Tacoma, Washington, where he practiced for two years. Shortly after he returned to San Fernando in 1955, he built a building for his practice with his sister Dr. Mary Oda and his brother Dr. Bo Sakaguchi. In addition to his service on many professional medical committees and serving as JAMA president, from 1973 to 1974, Marquette University honored Dr. Sakaguchi with their "Alumni Service Award for Professional Achievement and Distinguished Service" in 1975. His passions were big game fishing, judo, and UCLA sports. He once caught an 857-pound black marlin off the coast of Australia. He continued to practice until age 89.

GWENN M. JENSEN interviewed Dr. Sakaguchi on August 14, 2002, in San Fernando, CA.

SATO, Dr. William

GENERAL PRACTICE AND SURGERY

b. 1921 Carlsbad, CA
d. 2013, South Pasadena, CA

1942 Tulare Assembly Center, Gila River, health inspector

1944 (to 1946) Camp Blanding, 442d Regimental Combat Team, France, Po Valley, Leghorn, Lake Como, Italy. Awarded Combat Infantryman's Badge

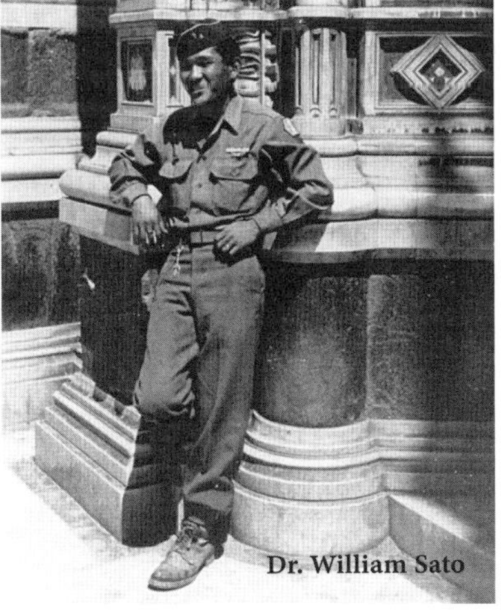
Dr. William Sato

1951 MD, Northwestern University Medical School, Chicago, IL

In 1941, at the time of Pearl Harbor, **Dr. William Sato** was in the pre-med program at UCLA. In May 1942, a train ride took him to Tulare Assembly Center where he and his wife Irene (Yoshikawa) spent their honeymoon. They were moved to Gila River in September where Sato worked as a health inspector. When his California draft board notified him that he was classified 4-C, or enemy alien, Sato wrote an angry letter of complaint. A week later, he was reclassified 1-A and drafted. He fought in Europe with the 442nd and served in the Occupation of Italy. When he returned to the United States, he went to medical school at Northwestern University graduating in 1951. A one-year internship at St. Luke's Hospital in Chicago and a surgical residency at the West Suburban Hospital located in Oak Park, Illinois, followed. The Satos' first son, William, was born at that time. Dr. Sato returned to Los Angeles in 1953 and spent one year practicing with Dr. Norman Kobayashi of Gardena. In October of that year, the Sato family welcomed a second son, David. In the spring of 1954, he opened his own practice in Little Tokyo and worked with the Japanese Hospital of Los Angeles that had been established by the early Issei in 1929. At the time, there were six other Nikkei MDs in Little Tokyo. In the early 1970s, he quit hospital practice and retired in 1997, after forty-four years of providing medical care to the community. Many people continued as his patients for his entire career.

Gwenn M. Jensen interviewed Dr. Sato on August 13, 2002, in South Pasadena, California.

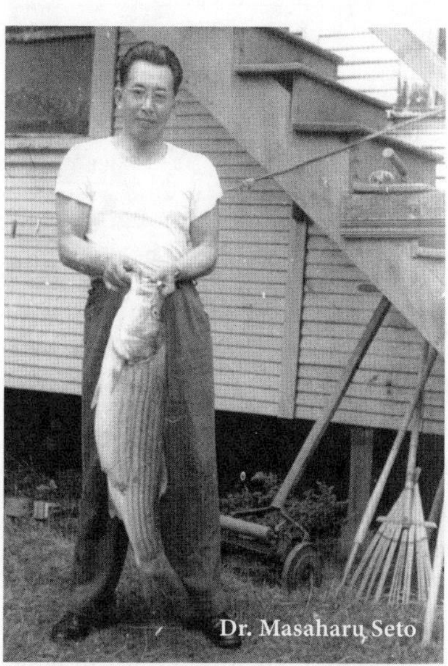
Dr. Masaharu Seto

SETO, Dr. Masaharu Richard

FAMILY PRACTITIONER
b. 1912 San Francisco, CA
d. 1985 Sacramento, CA

1941 MD, Marquette School of Medicine, Milwaukee, WI
1942 Internship and residency, Sacramento County Hospital and Yuba County Hospital, CA
Sacramento (Walerga) Assembly Center, Tule Lake, physician
1944 Residency, Silver Cross Hospital, Joliet, IL
1944 U.S. Army, Signal Corps, then 147th Medical Unit

Dr. Masa Seto delivered the first baby born at Tule Lake, Newell Kazuo Noda, on June 18, 1942. After leaving camp in mid-1943, he married Hideko "Deki" Nakazawa in Joliet, Illinois, where he had a residency. On December 31, 1944, the Army drafted Dr. Seto and eventually assigned him to the 147th Medical Unit until his transfer as Post Surgeon at Sand Island, Hawaii, caring for Okinawan prisoners of war. After his stint with the Army, "Doc" Seto returned to Sacramento in 1947 and established a family practice. Although he had no problems obtaining hospital privileges or re-establishing himself in the community, he did encounter difficulties obtaining malpractice insurance because the insurance companies felt a jury would not be fair to a doctor of Japanese heritage and declined to insure him. He finally obtained coverage from Lloyd's of London and practiced medicine for thirty-eight years, until his death. His wife "Deki" Sato, a UC Berkeley graduate, had an interesting career working as a medical social worker, first for the WCCA and later for WRA at Tule Lake.

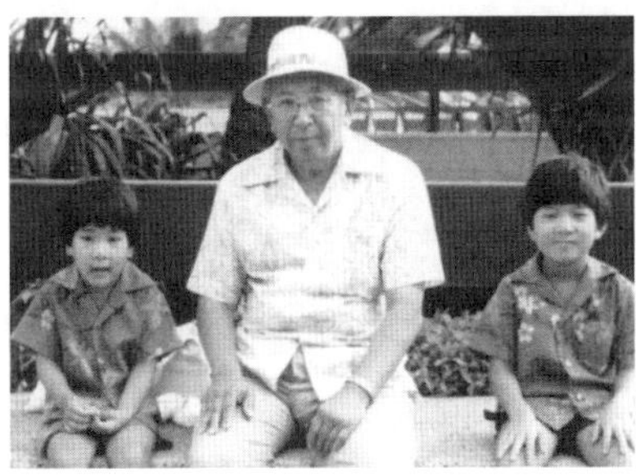

Interviewed by Paul Tsuneishi on November 26, 2002, in Sacramento, California, Mrs. H. Deki Seto also wrote responses to JAMA questions.

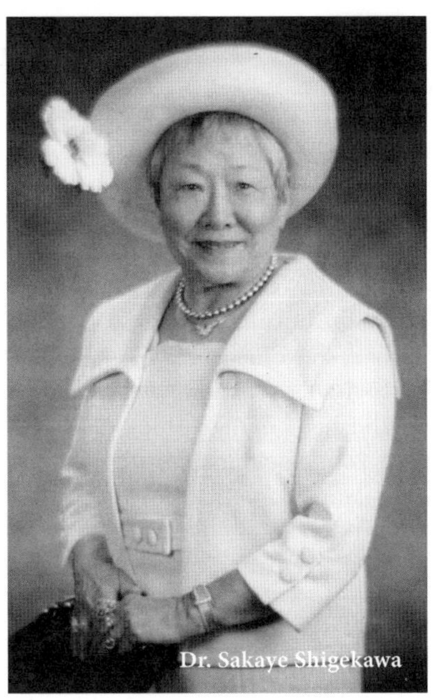

Dr. Sakaye Shigekawa

SHIGEKAWA, Dr. Sakaye

OBSTETRICIAN/GYNECOLOGIST

b. 1913 South Pasadena, CA
d. 2018 Los Angeles, CA

- 1940 MD, Loyola University Chicago Stritch School of Medicine, Chicago, IL
- 1941 Internship, Bay Regional Medical Center, Bay City, MI
  Started residency, L.A. County General Hospital, Los Angeles, CA
- 1942 Seaside Memorial Hospital, Terminal Island, CA
  Santa Anita Assembly Center, physician

After her internship, **Dr. Sakaye Shigekawa** began her obstetrics residency at L.A. County General Hospital, only to be dismissed in the wake of Pearl Harbor. She went to work at Seaside Memorial Hospital, a Navy facility in Long Beach, but that community was the first to be incarcerated. As one of seven doctors at Santa Anita Assembly Center, she helped care for seventeen thousand detainees. She left Santa Anita to complete her residency in Chicago at Walter Memorial Hospital. However, when the hospital cut her salary offer by half, she joined a local woman physician in her practice. A year later, she established her own office in an Irish and Polish neighborhood. She soon had a large practice in Chicago but found she did not like the climate. In 1948, she returned to Los Angeles to be near her family and started anew. Unlike Chicago, she encountered difficulty getting hospital privileges at area hospitals and practiced at the Japanese Hospital. After six months, she and an African American man became the first minority physicians accepted at Queen of Angels Hospital, and in 1977 she became the first woman elected president of the hospital's medical staff. Although she had a general practice, Dr. Shigekawa was in the delivery room every day, at least once and sometimes three to five times a day. She ended her obstetrics practice and hospital work in 1982. In her thirty-three years of obstetrics, she calculated that she delivered over twenty thousand babies, three generations, and never lost a mother.

GWENN M. JENSEN interviewed Dr. Shigekawa on August 19, 2002, in Los Angeles, California.

SUGIYAMA, Dr. Henry Iwao

OBSTETRICIAN/GYNECOLOGIST
b. 1914 Los Angeles, CA
d. 2012 Sacramento, CA

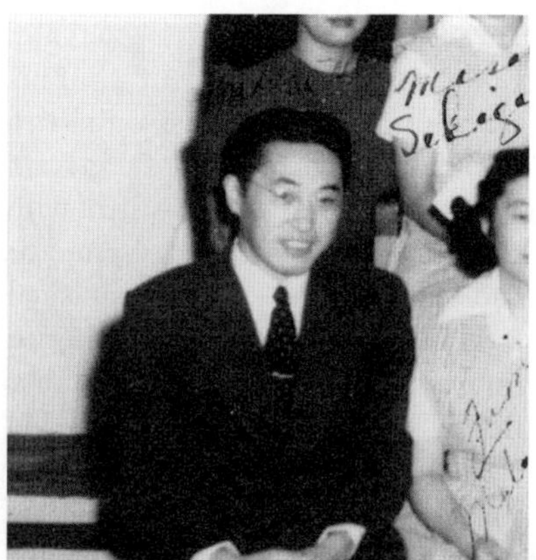

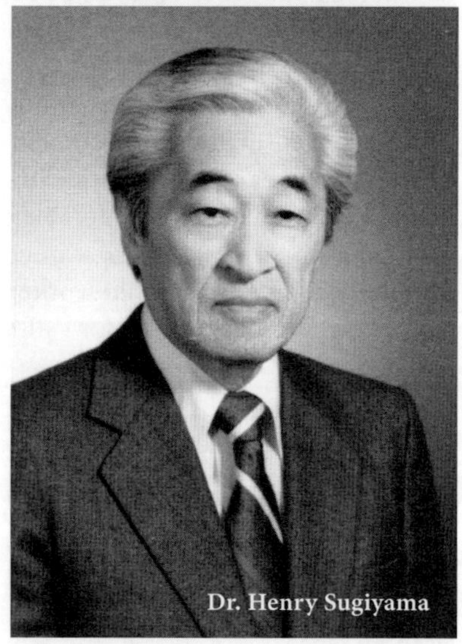

Dr. Henry Sugiyama

1941 MD, Marquette School of Medicine, Milwaukee, WI
Started internship at Sacramento County Hospital, CA
1942 Sacramento (Walerga) Assembly Center, Tule Lake, physician
1943 Topaz, physician

Initially, **Dr. Henry Sugiyama** went to Tule Lake but after it became a "Segregation Center" for "disloyals" (those who had answered "no-no" on questions 27 and 28 of the 1943 loyalty questionnaire), he and his family were sent to Topaz with their firstborn son. After the war ended, Dr. Sugiyama returned to Sacramento, set up a general and obstetrics practice, and had no trouble obtaining hospital privileges, first at Mercy Hospital and then at Sutter Maternity. He immediately had plenty of work from his former patients who remembered him from Tule Lake and Topaz. Some women continued to come from as far away as San Francisco to have him deliver their babies. When malpractice insurance skyrocketed for obstetricians in the 1970s, Dr. Sugiyama stopped delivering babies. Although he no longer did obstetrics, he continued a general private practice until he was seventy years old. In all, the Sugiyama family includes three sons, Ron, Alan, and Jon, and one stepson, Erik. When he retired in 1984, after thirty-nine years of providing medical care for his Sacramento patients, the community honored him with a special luncheon and "Dr. Henry I. Sugiyama Day."

GWENN M. JENSEN interviewed Dr. Sugiyama on August 31, 2002, in Sacramento, California.

SUZUKI, Dr. Masamichi "Mac"

OBSTETRICIAN/GYNECOLOGIST
b. 1918 Acampo, CA
d. 2014, Bloomfield Hills, MI

1939 Started University of California Medical School, San Francisco, CA
1942 Sacramento (Walerga) Assembly Center, Tule Lake, Minidoka, medical intern
1944 MD, Wayne State University School of Medicine, Detroit, MI
Internship and residency, Grace Hospital, Detroit, MI

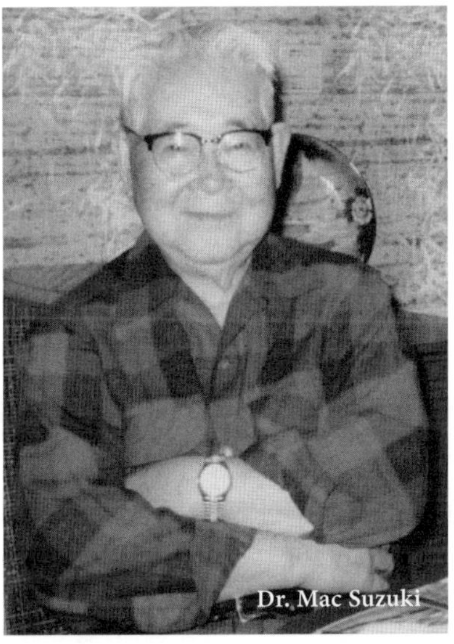
Dr. Mac Suzuki

Dr. Mac Suzuki was a third-year medical student when the war broke out. Sent to Walerga where he helped set up the clinic, he was moved to the hospital at Tule Lake where he worked essentially as an intern. Transferred to Minidoka for three short months, he left to finish his medical training at Wayne State University in Detroit, Michigan. After completing his residency, he went to work for the Atomic Bomb Casualty Commission and studied infertility in couples in Hiroshima. It was here that he met his future wife Wilma, a nurse, and they married upon their return to the U.S. Because she was Caucasian, they were turned away from the marriage bureau in Nevada and ended up marrying in Sacramento. Soon after, he visited with Dr. George Baba in Los Angeles, who was looking for a partner. But with his eyes burning from the smog, he decided he'd rather join a Detroit area group practice as an obstetrician/gynecologist. Drafted immediately, he spent the next two years as chief of OB/GYN at Shepard Air Force Base in Wichita Falls, Texas. Dr. Suzuki returned to the group practice and retired at the age of seventy-six. After first considering a career in pathology, he was pleased that circumstances changed his direction into women's health, a field he enjoyed fully.

GWENN M. JENSEN interviewed Dr. Suzuki on December 11, 2002, in Bloomfield Hills, Michigan.

TANAKA, Dr. Benjamin Masayoshi

GENERAL PRACTITIONER
b. 1887, Rappahoihoi, HI
d. 1975 Ontario, OR

1920 MD, University of Oregon Medical School, Portland, OR
1942 Santa Fe Internment Center, physician

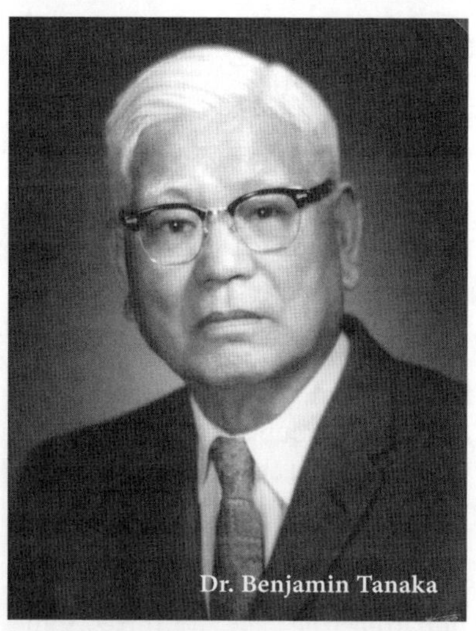
Dr. Benjamin Tanaka

Through the assistance of a *baishakunin* (go-between), **Dr. Ben Tanaka** married eighteen-year-old Michiye Yamada. He first practiced medicine in the Japanese district of Portland, Oregon, after earning his medical degree from the University of Oregon in 1920. His son "Gus" was born in 1923 and a daughter and second son followed soon thereafter. An avid golfer, he served as the first president of the Northwest Japanese Golf Association in 1931. Although a Hawaiʻian-born U.S. citizen, he had a difficult time documenting his citizenship. Because of this, during the war years, he was incarcerated at the Santa Fe INS camp as an enemy alien. As one of the few physicians at Santa Fe, the government kept him until he was one of the last internees to leave. When he returned to Portland after the war, the medical establishment turned its back on him. Not one hospital would grant him staff privileges. Invited by the local Issei and Nisei who had relocated to eastern Oregon just outside the Military Defense boundary, Dr. Tanaka moved to Ontario and opened a new practice. Dr. Tanaka continued to practice on a gradually reduced schedule until he was about eighty-four years old.

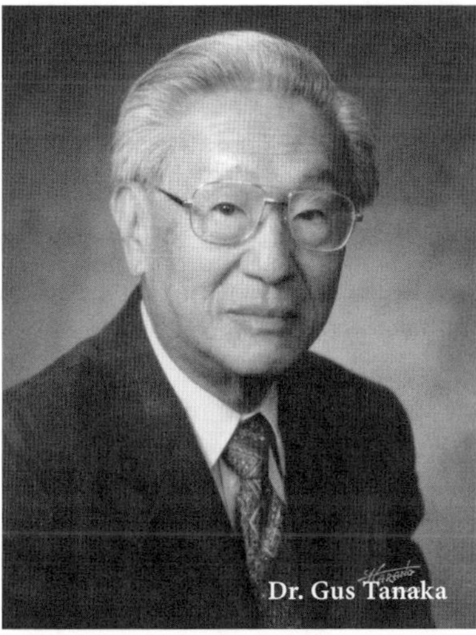

Dr. Gus Tanaka

TANAKA, Dr. Augustus "Gus" Masashi

GENERAL SURGEON
b. 1923, Portland, OR
d. 2015, Ontario, OR

1942 Portland Assembly Center, Minidoka, orderly
1951 MD, Long Island College of Medicine, Brooklyn, NY

Dr. Gus Tanaka left Reed College for Portland Assembly Center where he worked as an orderly for Drs. Robert Kinoshita and Robert Hajime Shiomi. After a brief transfer to Minidoka, he left to finish his premed at Haverford College, a Quaker school in Pennsylvania. Working on indigent patients during his internship at Kings County Hospital in New York, he developed tuberculosis and was hospitalized for months. His one-year straight surgical internship took two years to complete. During his residency, he met and married his wife Teddy (Teruko) Wada. They began their family immediately and all three children, Maja, John, and Susan, were born in Brooklyn. In 1958, when Dr. Tanaka was nearing the end of his five-year surgical residency at Kings County Hospital, his father, Dr. Ben Tanaka, asked him to join him in Ontario. Together, he and his father began the Tanaka Clinic. Dr. Tanaka maintained a surgical practice in Ontario from 1959, until his retirement in 1993. In addition to his medical duties, he served on the Oregon State Board of Health, the Oregon Board of Medical Examiners, and the Oregon Medical Professional Review Organization. He was also active in the Oregon Medical Association and served as president from 1971 to 1972. Over his career, he accumulated many honors including being named the outstanding physician of Oregon in 1993 among retirees.

GWENN M. JENSEN interviewed Dr. Tanaka on November 20, 2002, in Ontario, Oregon, about his life and the life of his father, Dr. Benjamin Masayoshi Tanaka.

THE TOGASAKI SISTERS

Kazue Togasaki, MD
OBSTETRICIAN
b. 1897 San Francisco, CA
d. 1992 Lafayette, CA

Mitsuye Togasaki Shida, RN
REGISTERED NURSE
b. 1902, San Francisco, CA
d. 1973 Honolulu, HI

Yoshiye Togasaki, MD
PUBLIC HEALTH PEDIATRICIAN
b. 1904, San Francisco, CA
d. 1999 Lafayette, CA

Chiye Togasaki Yamanaka, RN
REGISTERED NURSE
b. 1905, San Francisco, CA
d. 1990 Oakland, CA

Teru Togasaki, MD
GENERAL PRACTITIONER
b. 1907 San Francisco, CA
d. 1990 San Francisco, CA

Yaye Togasaki Breitenbach, RN
PSYCHIATRIC NURSE
b. 1908, San Francisco, CA
d. 2005 Oakland, CA

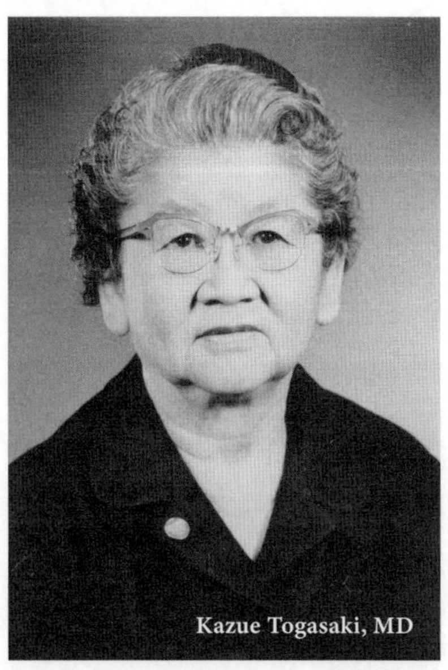
Kazue Togasaki, MD

Dr. Kazue Togasaki, the oldest of the Togasaki daughters, graduated from Stanford's Children's Hospital School of Nursing in 1924, and followed that in 1927, with a degree from the University of California School of Public Health Nursing. She worked for a while as a public health nurse but decided she wanted to be a doctor. In 1933, she and Megumi Shinoda became the first women of Japanese ancestry to receive medical degrees in the United States, Kazue from the Women's Medical College, Pennsylvania, and Megumi from Columbia. Kazue completed her internship at Children's Hospital of San Francisco, and in 1935, went into private practice until the war. Within days of arrival she was hard at work at Tanforan, then Tule Lake, and Manzanar. She left camp for an obstetrics residency at a Catholic hospital in Chicago. After the war, she reopened her obstetrics practice and was on staff at a number of hospitals in San Francisco. Devoted to her practice, she delivered over ten thousand babies, according to one count. She had a special interest in unwed mothers and even invited some of the more distressed to stay in her home. Her dedication and work in the community prompted the *San Francisco*

Examiner to name her one of the ten "Most Distinguished Women of 1970." She closed her practice when her memory began to fail. She suffered from Alzheimer's for more than twenty years before she died at the age of ninety-five.

After graduating from UC Berkeley about 1926, **Mitsuye Togasaki Shida, RN** received her nursing education from the nursing school at Children's Hospital in San Francisco. She married Chozo Shida, a widower from Hawai'i with two children, in 1934 and moved to Honolulu where she escaped the incarceration. During the war years, she worked as a public health nurse for the Palama Settlement, known as Honolulu's "Hull House," which provided public health programs to the community. For a time, she also worked for Issei physician, Dr. Harvey Saburo Hayashi, who was in private practice. When the first of her two daughters was born, she quit nursing and focused her energy on her children. Later she worked in the curio store the Shida family owned in Wahiawa and later their wholesale import business. Mitsuye spent her life as a nurse, mother, wife, and storeowner.

Once she earned her medical degree at Johns Hopkins in 1935, **Dr. Yoshiye Togasaki** became the second Nisei accepted as an intern at L.A. County General Hospital. Following this one-year rotating internship, she spent the next six years in a communicable disease residency at the hospital. She went into private practice for one year before the war started. As a specialist in public health, her expertise was put to use at Manzanar and Tule Lake. In 1943, she went to Bellevue Hospital in New York for a two-year pediatrics residency. After completing this residency, she went to Italy in 1946, for the U.N. Relief and Rehabilitation Administration, taking care of war refugees and Italian POWs. Upon her return, she went to work for the California State Health Department and, in 1951, joined Contra Costa County Health Department. As an early supporter of redress, she testified at the Commission on Wartime Relocation and Internment of Civilians hearings and urged others to present their stories as well. She retired from Contra Costa County as chief of preventive medical services and deputy health officer in 1972. Her retirement years were spent working for a variety of health and political causes. Before she died, the Diablo Valley JACL named a scholarship in her honor.

Chiye Togasaki Yamanaka, RN, obtained her nursing degree from the University of California at Berkeley in 1929, specializing in public health. She was incarcerated at Tanforan and Tule Lake with her sister Kazue. After leaving camp, she joined the Chicago City Health Department. When the war ended, she went to work for the San Francisco Visiting

Nurse Association and also worked as an obstetrics nurse. She later joined her husband, Tamezo, in Hiroshima, Japan, and was employed by the Atomic Energy Commission until 1959. At that time, care of her father and missionary work in Japan occupied her life until 1979. Chiye and her husband had one daughter, Sachiko. When sisters Kazue and Teru's health began to decline, Chiye returned from Japan to care for them.

Teru Togasaki, MD, received her medical degree from the University of California Medical School in 1936. Before the war, she had a thriving general practice in Sacramento, California. According to her nephew Gordon, Teru was the brightest of the Togasaki sisters and had a photographic memory. She was incarcerated at Poston with her brother Susumu and his family until she left to work as a resident physician in the tuberculosis unit of a New York City hospital. After the war, Teru decided not to return to her prewar general practice in Sacramento but practiced in Honolulu for thirteen years. She lived for a short time with her older sister Mitsuye and worked as a resident physician at the Salvation Army Boys' Home. In her clinical work, she became aware of the need for a new women's prison and worked tirelessly until it became a reality. Noted as the best diagnostician of the three sisters, Teru was characterized as "the epitome of the Hippocratic oath." In the mid-1960s, Teru returned to San Francisco and lived with her sister Kazue. She retired in 1972 but kept busy working with the League of Women Voters and other volunteer work.

Yaye Togasaki Breitenbach, RN, spent the war years in the armed services and was not incarcerated with the rest of the family. During her enlistment in the service, she worked in a battle fatigue unit, which led to her career in psychiatric nursing. She left the Army with the rank of colonel and joined the Veteran's Administration. One assignment led her to help set up the VA psychiatric hospital in Salt Lake City. She returned to New York where she married German photographer, Joseph Breitenbach.

GWENN M. JENSEN interviewed half-brother Shinobu and nephew Gordon Togasaki on September 3, 2002, in San Jose, California, and nephew David Togasaki on September 5, 2002, in Lafayette, California, about the lives of their sisters/aunts. Mary and Eizo Kobayashi interviewed Dr. Yoshiye Togasaki for the Diablo Valley JACL on March 27, 1993, and April 2, 6, and 9, 1994.

YAMAMOTO, Toshi (Yasutake)

PHYSICIAN'S ASSISTANT, BARBER

b. 1915 Seattle, WA
d. 2003 Los Angeles, CA

1942 Manzanar, vaccination program

After accompanying Dr. Yoshiye Togasaki to Manzanar, **Toshi Yamamoto** managed the vaccination

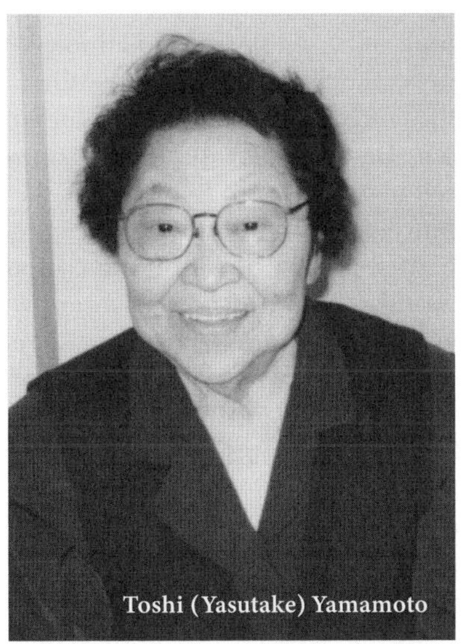
Toshi (Yasutake) Yamamoto

program. She left after one year to accompany her sixteen-year-old sister who had been awarded a college scholarship at the University of Chicago. While there, she worked for Vaughn's Seed Store. In her typical Don Quixote style, she applied at Vaughn's even though she had been told they would not hire people of Japanese ancestry. After the war, she returned to Los Angeles and became the first Japanese American to work at Bullock's Department Store. When several women protested her hiring, Bullock's management told them to accept Toshi or quit. On a Bullock's scholarship, Toshi trained to become a barber and eventually owned her own shop with her husband, George, also a barber. She met soon-to-be California Governor Reagan while working on his first campaign. When he won office, he selected Toshi to fill a position on the state Board of Barber Examiners, the first woman and ethnic minority appointed to it. She held this position until 2001 when she finally retired at the age of eighty-six. Toshi Yasutake Yamamoto was diagnosed with colon cancer two days after the JAMA interview. After months of treatment, she passed away on April 29, 2003, at the age of eighty-seven, in Los Angeles, California.

GWENN M. JENSEN interviewed Toshi Yamamoto on December 2, 2002, in Los Angeles, California.

YAMAZAKI, Dr. James N.

PEDIATRICIAN

b. 1916 Los Angeles, CA
d. 2021 White Salmon, WA

1943 MD, Marquette School of Medicine, Milwaukee, WI
1943 Internship, St. Louis City Hospital, St. Louis, MO
1944 U.S. Army, 106th Infantry Division, POW in Germany 1944-1945

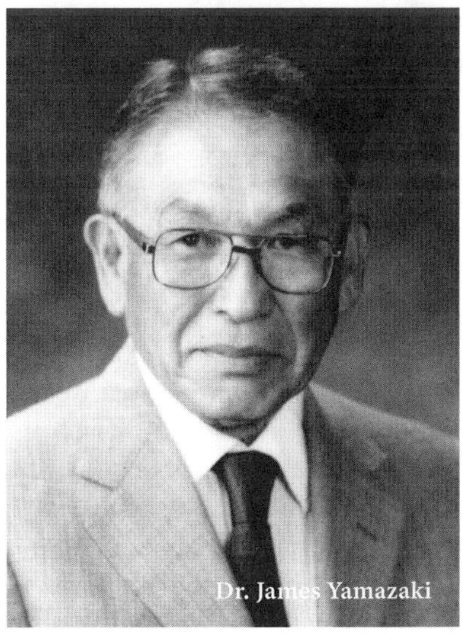
Dr. James Yamazaki

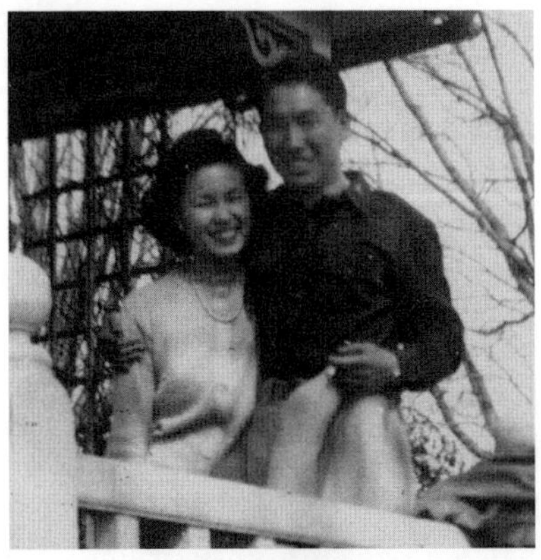

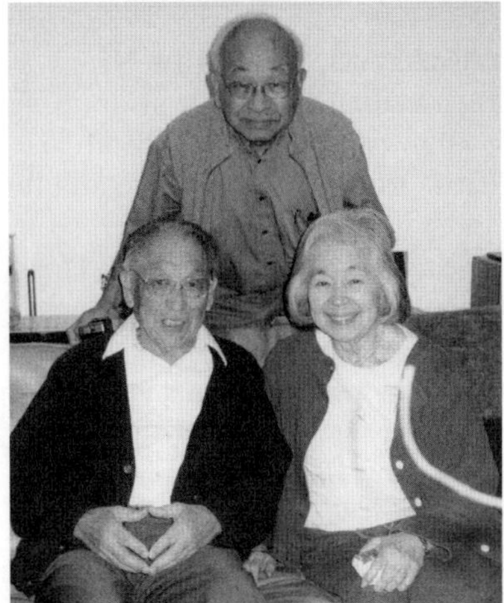

After graduation from UCLA, **Dr. James Yamazaki** attended medical school at Marquette and received his MD in 1943. By residing outside of the restricted military areas, he avoided incarceration. Because no Milwaukee hospital would accept a Nisei, even one with an Army commission, he interned at St. Louis City Hospital. In 1944, he received orders to report for active duty while working for the Chicago draft board, giving physicals to new recruits. A week before he left for training, he proposed, and he and Aki Hirashiki were married a month later. When the 106th Infantry Division shipped out, Dr. Yamazaki soon found himself in the midst of the Battle of the Bulge. Captured five days after the battle began, he spent the next six months as a German prisoner of war. After his discharge in 1946, he completed a pediatrics residency at Children's Hospital of Philadelphia, followed by another two-year residency at Children's Hospital of Cincinnati where his son, Paul, was born. Recruited by the Atomic Bomb Casualty Commission (ABCC) to study the impact of the atomic bomb on children, he worked in Nagasaki until 1951. Daughters Kathy and Carol were born after the family moved back to the States. Upon his return, Dr. Yamazaki taught and did research at UCLA for a year and opened his private pediatrics practice in 1953, in Los Angeles. Through the years, he has published numerous papers, written a memoir of his tenure with the ABCC, called *Children of the Atomic Bomb: An American Physician's Memoir of Nagasaki, Hiroshima, and the Marshall Islands* (Durham, NC: Duke University Press, 1995), and received many honors and awards. After his retirement in 1987 he participated in a documentary of his experiences in Nagasaki and taught an honors class at UCLA on "Nuclear Weapons: The Critical Decisions."

Paul Tsuneishi and Gwenn M. Jensen interviewed Dr. Yamazaki on December 3, 2002, in Van Nuys, California.

YASUI, Dr. Homer

GENERAL SURGEON
b. 1924, Hood River, OR
d. 2023, Portland, OR

1942 Orderly, sanitation inspector, Pinedale Assembly Center, orderly, Tule Lake
1949 MD, Hahnemann Medical School, Philadelphia, PA

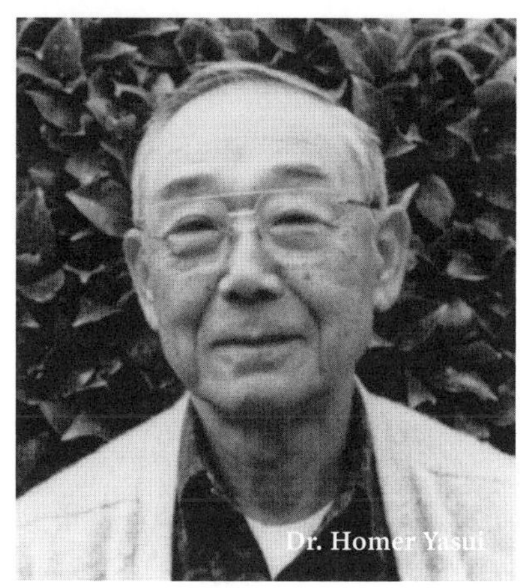

Dr. Homer Yasui

Dr. Homer Yasui left Tule Lake early, completed his education at the University of Denver, and went on to medical school at Hahnemann Medical School in Philadelphia. While in Philadelphia, he met his future wife, Miyuki (Miki) Yabe, and they were married in 1950, after his internship. As an intern, his preference for OB/GYN disappeared when he learned that most babies are born at night, so he decided to go into general surgery instead, influenced by his older brother Shu, who was a surgeon. Dr. Yasui completed his internship by the time he was twenty-five, but he felt that he was not ready for private practice. He applied for a general residency, which he described as being like a second year of internship, at Vassar Brothers Hospital in Poughkeepsie, New York. When he returned to Portland, he started a three-year surgical residency at Emanual Hospital, but his training was interrupted by the draft. He chose to serve in the Navy, and he and his wife and two daughters spent a year and a half in Iwakuni, Japan, where he served as an assistant medical officer. Once back in Portland, he applied for a residency at St. Vincent Hospital and finished his training. A son arrived in 1957 and completed the Yasui family. A year later, he opened a private surgical practice in Milwaukie, Oregon, a suburb of Portland. After nearly thirty years of practice, he retired in 1987.

GWENN M. JENSEN interviewed Dr. Yasui on July 23, 2002, in Portland, Oregon, and January 23, 2003.

Japanese Americal Medical Association (JAMA) Oral History Collection

While *Silent Scars of Healing Hands* uses only short excerpts from the JAMA oral history collection, we think you will appreciate the warmth and candor of each interviewee, as much as we, the interviewers, did. If you find you would like to read more of their stories, all JAMA interviews are archived and accessible in tape and transcript form at the Japanese American National Museum in Los Angeles.

ILLUSTRATIONS AND SOURCES

1. THE CALLING

p. 1 Dr. Murase, Murakami with nurses and doctors at the Poston concentration camp. Workers stand beside hospital barracks building. Six women, two men. Copyright held by the Japanese American National Museum (JANM).

9 Hospital scene at Topaz by Miné Okubo, courtesy of JANM (Gift of Miné Okubo Estate, 2007.62.161).

2. PREWAR MEDICAL TRAINING AND PRACTICES

11 Portrait of Dr. Katsumi J. Nakadate. Photo courtesy of James R. Nakadate.

14 Seto family portrait and Seto diploma courtesy of Mrs. Hideko Nakazawa Seto.

18 Photos courtesy of Mac Suzuki.

23 Photo courtesy of James R. Nakadate.

3. PEARL HARBOR

25 Byron, California. Farm families of Japanese ancestry boarding buses for Turlock Assembly center 65 miles away. An official of the Wartime Civil Control Administration is checking the families into the bus by number. Courtesy of the National Archives and Records Administration (NARA). https://ddr.densho.org/ddr-densho-151-143/

27 Photo courtesy of Mac Suzuki.

32 Photo courtesy of Dr. James N. Yamazaki.

37 Photo courtesy of James N. Yamazaki.

4. TEMPORARY DETENTION CENTERS

39 Oakland, California. Kimiko Kitagaki, young evacuee guarding the family baggage prior to departure by bus in one half hour to Tanforan Assembly Center. Her father was, until evacuation, in the cleaning and dyeing business. Courtesy of NARA. https://ddr.densho.org/ddr-densho-151-326/

48 Photo courtesy of NARA. https://ddr.densho.org/ddr-densho-151-56/

53 Newsletter courtesy of Karl Matsushita and the Japanese American National Library.

54 Evacuation instructions courtesy of Mrs. May Kambara.

5. ESTABLISHING CAMP HOSPITALS

57 Manzanar Relocation Center, Manzanar, California. Emergency hospital housed in temporary quarters at this War Relocation Authority center for evacuees of Japanese ancestry. Courtesy of NARA. https://ddr.densho.org/ddr-densho-151-70/

60 Photo courtesy of NARA. https://ddr.densho.org/ddr-densho-37-795/

63 Photo courtesy of NARA. https://ddr.densho.org/ddr-densho-151-475/

64 Tule Lake photo courtesy of Dr. Henry Sugiyama.

67 Ambulance photo courtesy of NARA. https://ddr.densho.org/ddr-densho-37-228/; Manzanar hospital photo courtesy of NARA. https://ddr.densho.org/ddr-densho-151-419/

70 Tule Lake group photo courtesy of Dr. Henry Sugiyama.

71 Dr. George Kambara letter courtesy of Mrs. May Kambara.

6. HELPING THE CAPTORS

73 Manzanar entrance photo courtesy of JANM.

76 Photos courtesy of JANM.

7. A TIME TO IMPROVISE

79 Jerome Relocation Center, Denson,

Arkansas. A former Californian, Doctor Fugikawa, examining a patient, S. Ego, in the center hospital fluroscope. Courtesy of NARA. https://ddr.densho.org/ddr-densho-37-627/

83 Photo courtesy of JANM.

85 Photos courtesy of JANM.

8. CAMARADERIE, RIVALRIES, AND CONFLICT

87 Photo courtesy of JANM.

91 Photo courtesy NARA. https://ddr.densho.org/ddr-densho-37-805/

92 Photo courtesy of JANM.

9. RIOTS AND SEGREGATION

95 Photo courtesy of JANM.

101 Photo courtesy of Dr. Henry Sugiyama

10. VISITORS FROM THE OUTSIDE

105 Miné Okubo illustration courtesy of JANM.

11. EARLY EXITS TO THE OUTSIDE

111 Sacramento Assembly Center: Masamichi Suzuki is leaves his barrack room at the Assembly center. He has had three years of advanced education which includes three years at the University of California Medical School and is a member of Phi Beta Kappa. He has been assisting in the Assembly center hospital and hopes later to specialize in pathology. Courtesy of NARA. https://ddr.densho.org/ddr-densho-151-277/

115 Photo courtesy of NARA. https://ddr.densho.org/ddr-densho-93-16/

12. "I AM PROUD TO SERVE"

117 Dr. and Mrs. Masaharu Seto taken in Chicago, after wedding on June 25, 1943, before Masaharu left for military duty. Photo courtesy of Mrs. Hideko Nakazawa Seto.

122 Photo courtesy of Dr. James N. Yamazaki.

123 Photo courtesy of Dr. James N. Yamazaki.

127 Photo courtesy of James R. Nakadate.

129 (1) Charcoal illustration of Dr. Katsumi James Nakadate courtesy of James R. Nakadate; (2) photo courtesy of Dr. Mary Oda; (3) armored vehicle photo courtesy of Dr. William Sato.

13. LAST DAYS OF CAMP

133 Original WRA caption: *Shaved heads, but not shaved faces, were required of the Hokoku as is evidenced by this "alien enemy" sent to Santa Fe Internment Camp June 24, 1945 with 399 other pro-Japan agitators.* Courtesy of NARA. https://ddr.densho.org/ddr-densho-37-186/

136 Photo courtesy of Dr. Henry Sugiyama

137 Courtesy of NARA. https://ddr.densho.org/ddr-densho-37-422/

14. RESETTLEMENT AND RETURN TO THE WEST COAST

139 Closing of the Jerome Relocation Center, Denson, Arkansas. Jerome residents with their hand luggage wait at the chair car entrance for their names to be called by the War Relocation Authority official checking the list. Courtesy of NARA. https://ddr.densho.org/ddr-densho-37-616/

141 Photo courtesy of Dr. Homer Yasui.

143 Photo courtesy of Dr. William Sato.

144 Photo courtesy of NARA. https://ddr.densho.org/ddr-densho-37-430/

145 Photo courtesy of Dr. Sakaye Shigekawa.

147 Photo courtesy of Dr. Sanbo Sakaguchi.

EPILOGUE

153 Photo courtesy of Dr. Henry Sugiyama.

155 Photos courtesy of Dr. Henry Sugiyama.

156 Photo courtesy of Gwenn Jensen.

158 Photo courtesy of Dr. Shigeru Hara

161 Photo courtesy of Gwenn Jensen.

162 Photos courtesy of James R. Nakadate.

164 Photo courtesy of Dr. Mary Oda.

165 (1) Photo courtesy of Dr. Sanbo Sakaguchi; (2) photo courtesy of Dr. William Sato.

166 Photo courtesy of Mrs. Hideko Nakazawa Seto.

167 (1) Photo courtesy of Mrs. Hideko Nakazawa Seto; (2) photo courtesy of Dr. Sakaye Shigekawa.

168 Photos courtesy of Dr. Henry Sugiyama.

169 Photo courtesy of Gwenn Jensen.

170 Photo courtesy of Dr. Gus Tanaka.

171 Photo courtesy of Dr. Gus Tanaka.

172 Photo courtesy of David Togasaki.

175 (1) Photo courtesy of Gwenn Jensen; (2) Photo courtesy of Dr. James N. Yamazaki.

176 Photos courtesy of Dr. James N. Yamazaki.

177 Photo courtesy of Dr. Homer Yasui.

REFERENCES AND NOTES

INTRODUCTION

Commission on Wartime Relocation and Internment of Civilians. *Personal Justice Denied.* Washington, D.C.: The Civil Liberties Public Education Fund; Seattle: University of Washington Press, 1997. [Originally published by the U.S. Government Printing Office in 1982 and 1983.]

Daniels, Roger. *Prisoners Without Trial: Japanese Americans in World War II.* New York: Hill and Wang, 1993.

Dempster, Brian Komei, ed. *From Our Side of the Fence: Growing Up in America's Concentration Camps.* San Francisco: Japanese Cultural and Community Center of Northern California, 2001.

Fiset, Louis. *Imprisoned Apart: The World War II Correspondence of an Issei Couple.* Seattle: University of Washington Press, 1997.

______. "The Heart Mountain Hospital Strike of June 24, 1943." In *Remembering Heart Mountain.* Edited by Mike Mackey. Powell, WY: Western History Publications, 1998.

______. "Public Health in World War II Assembly Centers for Japanese Americans." *Bulletin of the History of Medicine* 73 (1999): 565–84.

______. "Licensed Nikkei MDs WWII Era, All Physicians in USA." Unpublished compilation, 2002.

______. "Medical Care for Interned Enemy Aliens: A Role for the U.S. Public Health Service in World War II." *American Journal of Public Health* 93, no. 10 (2003).

Gutierrez, Michelle. "Medical Mystique: Medical Care at the Manzanar War Relocation Center." Unpublished paper, California State University, Fullerton, 1986.

______. "Medicine in a Crisis Situation: The Effect of Culture on Health Care in the World War II Japanese American Detention Camps." MA thesis, California State University, Fullerton, 1989.

Hansen, Arthur A., ed. *Japanese American World War II Evacuation Oral History Project.* Vol. 1: *Internees.* Westport, CT: Meckler, 1991.

______. *Japanese American World War II Evacuation Oral History Project.* Vol. 2: *Administrators.* Westport, CT: Meckler, 1991.

Hirabayashi, Lane Ryo. *The Politics of Fieldwork: Research in an American Concentration Camp.* Tucson: University of Arizona Press, 1999.

Hirahara, Naomi. "Forever Young: The Akita Sisters of L.A." *Rafu Magazine,* December 17, 1994.

______. *An American Son: The Story of George Aratani, Founder of Mikasa and Kenwood.* Los Angeles: Japanese American National Museum, 2001.

______. *A Taste of Strawberries: The Independent Journey of Nisei Farmer Manabi Hirasaki.* Los Angeles: Japanese American National Museum, 2003.

______. *A Scent of Flowers: The Southern California Flower Market and Its Multicultural Community, 1912–2000.* Los Angeles: Southern California Flower Growers, Inc., 2004.

Iwasaki, Pamela. "'We Must Endure...': A Look at Health Care in the Japanese American

Internment Camps." Unpublished paper, School of Medicine, University of California, San Diego, 1989.

Jensen, Gwendolyn M. "The Experience of Injustice: Health Consequences of the Japanese American Internment." PhD diss., University of Colorado at Boulder, 1997.

Kaji, Troy Tashiro. "City View Hospital and the Japanese Hospitals of California." Fellowship Report, School of Medicine, University of California, Davis, 1986.

_______. "Not the Yellow Peril: The Japanese-American Physicians of California, 1887–1945." Unpublished manuscript, 2001.

Kikuchi, Julie Sumie. "'The Tuberculosis Problem': A Quiet Legacy of the Japanese-American Internment Camps." Honors paper, Stanford University, 1995.

Kurahara, Jan. *Ganbatte.* Bloomington, IN: 1st Books, 1999.

Mackey, Mike. *Heart Mountain: Life in Wyoming's Concentration Camp.* Powell, WY: Western History Publications, 2000.

McKay, Susan. *The Courage Our Stories Tell: The Daily Lives and Maternal Child Health Care of Japanese American Women at Heart Mountain.* Powell, WY: Western History Publications, 2002.

Nakano, Mei T. *Japanese American Women: Three Generations, 1890–1990.* Berkeley, CA: Mina Press Publishing; San Francisco: National Japanese American Historical Society, 1990.

Niiya, Brian, ed. *Japanese American History: An A-to-Z Reference from 1868 to the Present.* New York: Facts on File, Inc., 1993.

Nishimoto, Richard S., and Lane Ryo Hirabayashi, eds. *Inside an American Concentration Camp: Japanese American Resistance at Poston, Arizona.* Tucson: University of Arizona Press, 1995.

Shirai, Noboru. *Tule Lake: An Issei Memoir.* English ed. Sacramento, CA: Muteki Press, 2001.

Smith, Susan L. "Caregiving in Camp: Japanese American Women and Community Health in World War II." In *Guilt By Association: Essays on Japanese Settlement, Internment, and Relocation in the Rocky Mountain West.* Edited by Mike Mackey. Powell, WY: Western History Publications, 1978.

Weglyn, Michi. *Years of Infamy: The Untold Story of America's Concentration Camps.* New York: Morrow Quill Paperbacks, 1976.

Worthen, Dennis. "Nisei Pharmacists in World War II." *Pharmacy in History* 45 (2003): 58–65.

Yamamoto, Fusako. "The Togasaki Family: Remarkable Pioneers."

Pacific Citizen (Holiday Issue), December 2002.

1. THE CALLING

Japanese American Medical Association (JAMA) interviews with Shigeru Hara, Masako (Kusayanagi) Miura, Mary (Sakaguchi) Oda, William Sato, Sakaye Shigekawa, Augustus "Gus" Masashi Tanaka, and Gordon and Shinobu Togasaki.

Kobayashi, Mary and Eizo (Diablo Valley Japanese American Citizens League [JACL]). Interview with Dr. Yoshiye Togasaki, March 27, 1993; April 2, 6, and 9, 1994.

2. PREWAR MEDICAL TRAINING AND PRACTICES

Fiset, "Licensed Nikkei MDs WWII Era" (see Introduction).

Hirahara, Naomi. Interview with Y. Fred Fujikawa, April 1, 1989.

JAMA interviews with Hara, Richard Kinoshita, Katsumi James Nakadate, Oda, Sanbo Sakaguchi, Hideko "Deki" Nakazawa Seto, Shigekawa, Henry Iwao Sugiyama, Masamichi "Mac" Suzuki, and James N. Yamazaki.

3. PEARL HARBOR

Immediately after the bombing of Pearl Harbor on December 7, 1941, the FBI began to round up Japanese community leaders and other prominent resident aliens, now deemed "enemy aliens," and hold them in temporary detention sites such as county jails. Some were released, but most were transferred to seven internment camps or the more than two dozen temporary camps run by the Immigration and Naturalization Service (INS) under the authority of the Department of Justice; others were incarcerated in prisons run by the Army. Surprisingly, there is no complete list of all of these sites. However, the permanent INS alien internment locations were: Fort Lincoln, near Bismarck, North Dakota; Fort Missoula, Montana; Fort Stanton, south of Ruidoso, and Santa Fe, New Mexico; and Crystal City, Kenedy, and Segoville, near Dallas, Texas.

Hansen, Arthur A. Interview with Frank F. Chuman (Oral History #1521). Fullerton: Japanese American Project of the Oral History Program at California State University, Fullerton, 1975.

JAMA interviews with Frank F. Chuman, Hara, Kinoshita, Miura, Nakadate, Seto, Sugiyama, Suzuki, Tanaka, Toshi Yamamoto, and Yamazaki.

4. TEMPORARY DETENTION CENTERS

Initially people were incarcerated in sixteen temporary sites that the government euphemistically called "Assembly Centers." Today many people refer to them as "temporary detention," call them by their common name, or by the government's term, "assembly center." We have chosen to use all of those terms, especially using the terms that interviewees reference. All, except as noted, were located in California: Fresno; Marysville (commonly known as Arboga); Mayer (in Arizona); Merced; Owens Valley; Pinedale (near Fresno); Pomona; Portland (in Oregon); Puyallup (in Washington); Sacramento (also known as Walerga); Salinas; Santa Anita (near Los Angeles); Stockton; Tanforan (near San Francisco); Tulare; and Turlock.

Hansen interview with Chuman (see Chapter 3).

Hirahara, Naomi. Interviews with Fujikawa (see Chapter 2) and Robert Toshio Obi, June 20, 1990.

JAMA interviews with Emi (Somekawa) Beckwith, Chuman, Hara, Miura, Sato, Shigekawa, Sugiyama, Suzuki, Yamamoto, and Homer Yasui.

Kobayashi, Mary and Eizo (Diablo Valley JACL). Interview with Dr. Yoshiye Togasaki, March 27, 1993; April 2, 6, and 9, 1994.

Unrau, Harlan D. "Chapter Ten: Operation of Manzanar War Relocation Center March–December, 1942." In *The Evacuation and Relocation of Persons of Japanese Ancestry During World War: II: A Historical Study of the Manzanar War Relocation Center.* Washington, D.C.: United States Department of the Interior/National Park Service, 1996.

______. "Chapter Twelve: Operation of Manzanar War Relocation Center, January 1943–1945." In *The Evacuation and Relocation of Persons of Japanese Ancestry During World War II: A Historical Study of the Manzanar War Relocation Center.* Washington, D.C.: United States Department of the Interior/National Park Service, 1996.

5. ESTABLISHING CAMP HOSPITALS

More than 110,000 people were incarcerated in ten permanent detention facilities that the government called "Relocation Centers": in California, Tule Lake and Manzanar; in Arizona, Poston (officially called Colorado River) and Gila River; Topaz (officially named Central Utah), Utah; Minidoka, Idaho; Heart Mountain, Wyoming; Amache (officially Granada), Colorado; and in Arkansas, Jerome and Rohwer. Many times, interviewees and others refer to these centers as "internment camps" or just "camp." While the only true internment camps were those operated by the INS that imprisoned people classified as enemy aliens, many people refer to the imprisonment of Japanese Americans as "the internment" and the sites as "internment camps" or just "camp." While recognizing these facilities were concentration camps, we have referred to them by their official name as well as the commonly used terms, especially those used by interviewees.

JAMA interviews with Beckwith, Hara, Iwao George Kawakami, Kinoshita, Miura, Oda, Sugiyama, and Suzuki.

Mamiya Medical Heritage Center. "Benjamin Makoto Higashi." In *In Memoriam—Doctors of Hawai'i* 1986. http://hml.org/mmhc/mdindex/ higashi.html (accessed 21 October 2002).

Tsuneishi, Paul. Interview with Joe Yamakido, November 25, 2002. Archived at the Japanese American National Museum, Los Angeles.

U.S. Bureau of the Census. *Statistics of the United States, Colonial Times to 1957: A Statistical*

Abstract Supplement. Washington, D.C.: Government Printing Office, 1960.

6. HELPING THE CAPTORS

JAMA interviews with Hara, Tanaka, and Yasui.

7. A TIME TO IMPROVISE

Hirahara interview with Fujikawa (see Chapter 2).

JAMA interviews with Hara, Miura, Sugiyama, Suzuki, and Tanaka.

Jensen, Gwenn M. "System Failure: Health-Care Deficiencies in the World War II Japanese American Detention Centers." *Bulletin of the History of Medicine* 73 (1999): 602–28.

8. CAMARADERIE, RIVALRIES, AND CONFLICT

Hirahara interview with Fujikawa (see Chapter 2).

JAMA interviews with Hara, Suzuki, and Yamamoto.

9. RIOTS AND SEGREGATION

Hansen, Arthur A., and David A. Hacker. "The Manzanar Riot: An Ethnic Perspective." *Amerasia Journal* 2, no. 2 (1974): 112–57.

Hansen interview with Chuman (see Chapter 3).

JAMA interviews with Chuman, Miura, and Suzuki. Kobayashi interview with Y. Togasaki (see Chapter 4).

Shirai, Eucaly A. "JAMA project," 18 October 2002, personal email to Gwenn Jensen.

War Relocation Authority. "Tule Lake Incident, Report on the Beating of Dr. Reece M. Pedicord, November 1, 1943." From the personal research collection of Eucaly A. Shirai. Also available from the National Archives, Record Group 210, Washington, D.C.; and Japanese American

Evacuation and Resettlement Records, Bancroft Library, University of California, Berkeley.

10. VISITORS FROM THE OUTSIDE

JAMA interviews with Sakaguchi and Yamazaki.

11. EARLY EXITS TO THE OUTSIDE

JAMA interviews with Sato, Shigekawa, and Yasui.

Kessler, Lauren. *Stubborn Twig: Three Generations in the Life of a Japanese American Family.* New York: Random House, 1993.

12. "I AM PROUD TO SERVE"

JAMA interviews with Kinoshita, Nakadate, Tanaka, and Yamazaki.

Kobayashi interview with Y. Togasaki (see Chapter 4).

13. LAST DAYS OF CAMP

JAMA interviews with George Taro Akamatsu, Beckwith, Miura, and Sugiyama.

14. RESETTLEMENT AND RETURN TO THE WEST COAST

Davila, Florangela. "Town Opened Doors for War's Outcasts." *Seattle Times,* February 17, 2002.

JAMA interviews with Akamatsu, Kinoshita, Oda, Sakaguchi, Sato, Shigekawa, Tanaka, G. and S. Togasaki, and Yasui.

EPILOGUE

Chuman, Frank F. *The Bamboo People: The Law and Japanese-Americans.* Del Mar, CA: Publisher's Inc., 1976.

Hashimoto, Mas. "Dr. K: A Doctor to Nikkei Internees." *Pacific Citizen* (Holiday Issue), December 2000.

Nakadate, Neil. "On Being a Doctor: Doctor's Luck." *Annals of Internal Medicine* 137 (2002): 142.

About JANM

The mission of the Japanese American National Museum is to promote understanding and appreciation of America's ethnic and cultural diversity by sharing the Japanese American experience.

As the national repository of Japanese American history, JANM creates groundbreaking historical and arts exhibitions, educational public programs, award-winning documentaries, and innovative curriculum that illuminate the stories and the rich cultural heritage of people of Japanese ancestry in the United States. JANM also speaks out when diversity, individual dignity and social justice are undermined, vigilantly sharing the hard-fought lessons accrued from this history.

JANM has the extraordinary privilege and responsibility of preserving and sharing the stories of more than 125,000 people of Japanese descent who were incarcerated in America's concentration camps. The reprinting of *Silent Scars of Healing Hands* coincides with today's mass detention of immigrants who are subject to poor conditions and healthcare in government facilities. JANM is unwavering in our mission—to tell the full story of the Japanese American community, both its struggles and triumphs, to stand firmly and unapologetically in defense of truth and justice. In doing so, we proudly stand true to our mission and honor the legacy of generations who came before us.

About JAMA

The Japanese American Medical Association (JAMA), composed of about 175 members representing more than 55 specialties, is dedicated to the care of patients in Southern California, primarily in Los Angeles, Orange, and Riverside counties. Since its founding in 1947, JAMA has grown to reflect its members and their achievements. The organization initially served as a professional and social setting for its members and families during the postwar era at a time when hospital privileges were generally inaccessible to Japanese American physicians.

While JAMA today continues to provide a venue for socializing and professional networking, the organization has in recent years expanded to meet the needs and challenges of its members. In addition to an annual gathering to introduce members to physicians-in-training in the area, JAMA initiated a mentor program to help guide these young professionals in their selected specialties in the community. Moreover, JAMA attained tax-exempt status as a charitable organization and established a Scholarship Fund for deserving medical students. Finally, JAMA is proud to be part of the history of this publication, *Silent Scars of Healing Hands,* which relates the experiences of Nisei medical providers who were incarcerated during World War II (some of them were JAMA members).

JAMA continues to serve the community and recognizes its individual members who donate their time and services to promote health care excellence.